STATISTICS AND DATA ANALYTICS

FOR HEALTH DATA MANAGEMENT

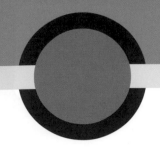

CONTENTS

STATISTICS AND DATA ANALYTICS
FOR HEALTH DATA MANAGEMENT

Nadinia Davis
MBA, RHIA, CHDA, CCS, FAHIMA

Program Coordinator
Health Information Management
Delaware Technical Community College
Wilmington, Delaware

Betsy Shiland
MS, RHIA, CHDA, CPHQ, CPC, CCS, CPB, CTR

AHIMA Approved ICD-10-CM/PCS Trainer
Former Assistant Professor
Allied Health Department
Community College of Philadelphia
Philadelphia, Pennsylvania

ELSEVIER

ELSEVIER

3251 Riverport Lane
St. Louis, Missouri 63043

STATISTICS AND DATA ANALYTICS FOR HEALTH DATA MANAGEMENT   ISBN: 978-1-4557-5315-4

Notices

Knowledge and best practice in this field are constantly changing. As new research and experience broaden our understanding, changes in research methods, professional practices, or medical treatment may become necessary.

Practitioners and researchers must always rely on their own experience and knowledge in evaluating and using any information, methods, compounds, or experiments described herein. In using such information or methods they should be mindful of their own safety and the safety of others, including parties for whom they have a professional responsibility.

With respect to any drug or pharmaceutical products identified, readers are advised to check the most current information provided (i) on procedures featured or (ii) by the manufacturer of each product to be administered, to verify the recommended dose or formula, the method and duration of administration, and contraindications. It is the responsibility of practitioners, relying on their own experience and knowledge of their patients, to make diagnoses, to determine dosages and the best treatment for each individual patient, and to take all appropriate safety precautions.

To the fullest extent of the law, neither the Publisher nor the authors, contributors, or editors, assume any liability for any injury and/or damage to persons or property as a matter of products liability, negligence or otherwise, or from any use or operation of any methods, products, instructions, or ideas contained in the material herein.

International Standard Book Number: 978-1-4557-5315-4

Senior Content Strategist: Linda Woodard
Content Development Manager: Luke Held
Senior Content Development Specialist: Diane Chatman
Publishing Services Manager: Julie Eddy
Project Manager: Mike Sheets
Design Direction: Renée Duenow

Printed in China

Last digit is the print number: 9 8 7 6 5 4 3 2 1

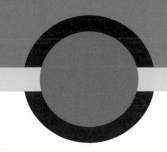

CONTRIBUTOR AND REVIEWERS

CONTRIBUTOR

Alice M. Noblin, PhD, RHIA, CCS
Health Informatics and Information Management
Undergraduate Program Director and Assistant Professor
Department of Health Management & Informatics
University of Central Florida
Orlando, Florida

REVIEWERS

Lisa Cerrato, MS, RHIA
Coordinator and Professor
Department of Health Information Management and Technology
Columbus State Community College
Columbus, Ohio

Angela Campbell, RHIA, AHIMA
Medical Insurance Manager
Eastern Illinois University
Charleston, Illinois

Pat DeVoy, EdS, LPN, RHIT, CMA (AAMA)
Faculty
Davenport University
Warren, Michigan

Marsha Dolan, MBA, RHIA, FAHIMA
Coordinator, Health Informatics and Information Management
Missouri Western State University
St. Joseph, Missouri

Alice M. Noblin, PhD, RHIA, CCS
Health Informatics and Information Management
Undergraduate Program Director and Assistant Professor
Department of Health Management & Informatics
University of Central Florida
Orlando, Florida

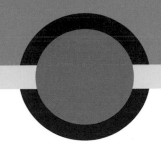

PREFACE

Today, the work of the health information management (HIM) professional positively impacts patient health and well-being at every stage of health care delivery. From their early days as organizers of paper charts in the hospital basement, these professionals are now facilitators of health data, serving as the bridge among clinicians, administrators, regulators, researchers, payers, and of course, patients. Health information professionals are no longer mere collectors of patient data but are called upon to manage, analyze, and present health data to each of these stakeholders. As stewards of this data and the statistics generated from it, HIM professionals have become central to the delivery of patient care in every health care setting.

Statistics and Data Analytics for Health Data Management was written with precisely this important new role in mind. First, this text acknowledges the novelty of the HIM professional as an analyst of data, and it offers an engaging, student-centered approach to the often daunting subject of statistics. Using a friendly tone and a colorful design, this book welcomes all students entering this field, even those with limited mathematical skills. It offers illustrations and plenty of real-world examples to take otherwise abstract statistical concepts and ground them in a way students can understand. Second, *Statistics and Data Analytics for Health Data Management* recognizes that many students enter an HIT or HIM program with limited experience in a clinical setting. To that end, the text provides ample visuals and descriptions that aim to increase the reader's familiarity with a variety of health care settings. The goal is to make the connection for students, at every level, between health data, statistics, and their purpose: improving the care of the patient.

As such, *Statistics and Data Analytics for Health Data Management* emphasizes the practical use of data. Everywhere possible, this text takes statistical concepts and shows their application in the workplace. The scope of the book is designed to satisfy the statistics competencies for the RHIT and RHIA exams, and it will serve as an onramp for individuals planning to sit for the Certified Health Data Analyst (CHDA) exam. With its focus on practical application, however, *Statistics and Data Analytics for Health Data Management* is not written solely for the classroom, but also as a professional resource. Because there is a wealth of practical advice in the text, HIM practitioners can refer to the instructions and immediately apply them to a problem at hand.

KEY FEATURES

Statistics and Data Analytics for Health Data Management offers an accessible, easy-to-understand text, and it includes several features to aid student comprehension. Throughout each chapter, it includes Takeaway boxes that highlight key points and important concepts. Intra-text exercises generally follow each main heading, giving students time to pause, reflect, and retain what they have learned. A Stat Tip feature explains trickier calculations and warns of pitfalls, and a Math Review box reminds students of the basic arithmetic, often with additional practice.

Each chapter opens with learning objectives and key terms, and the book breaks the definitions of the key terms into the margins for easy understanding. The margins also spell out commonly used acronyms for quick reference. The chapters finish with Review Questions tied to each learning objective, allowing students to check their understanding of all aspects of the topic.

To strengthen this book's hands-on, practical approach, every chapter includes a series of Brief Cases—scenarios drawn from the real work on the job. These case studies have been woven through the chapters, taking the information presented and applying it to situations encountered by HIM professionals every day. Each Brief Case includes an activity, giving the student the opportunity to practice newly acquired skills in a professional situation.

The appendices have answers to the Brief Case scenarios and all the intra-text exercises and Review Questions in the text. In addition, every formula that appears throughout *Statistics and Data Analytics for Health Data Management* has been listed separately at the back of the book for easy reference.

ORGANIZATION OF THE TEXT

Unit 1 imparts the basics of statistics and data analytics, with Chapter 1 focusing on the importance of data, statistics, and its uses and users in health care. Chapter 2 reviews each mathematical concept used in the book as a whole, giving some students the skills needed to work through the text and others a reminder of the arithmetic they learned long ago. Chapter 3 is dedicated to data presentation—the tables, charts, and graphs working HIM professionals use to communicate their findings.

Unit 2 introduces the practical application of statistics and data analysis in various health care settings, both inpatient and outpatient. In Chapters 4 through 6, students learn to calculate all the most important stats—working with patient encounters, occupancy and LOS, morbidity, mortality, and other rates, including public health statistics, like natality and mortality rates—just to name a few. Chapter 7 details the statistics used within the HIM department, measuring productivity, reimbursement, and compliance, while Chapter 8 introduces the calculations used for budgeting.

The final section, Unit 3, provides the background on more advanced data analysis concepts: data scrubbing and mapping and inferential statistics.

ONLINE RESOURCES FOR THE INSTRUCTOR

The TEACH Instructor's Resource Manual provides detailed lesson plans, PowerPoints, classroom handouts, and an Examview test bank. The lesson plans allow instructors to quickly familiarize themselves with the material in each chapter. PowerPoints are tailored to each lesson, highlighting the most important concepts from the text. The Examview test bank includes over 500 questions. Each question is tied to a specific objective and Bloom's taxonomy.

Instructors using this textbook also have access to a full suite of course management tools on Evolve. The Evolve Website may be used to publish the class syllabus, outlines, and lecture notes. Instructors can set up e-mail communication and virtual office hours and engage the class using discussion boards and chat rooms. An online class calendar is available to share important dates and other information.

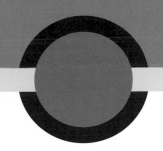

DETAILED CONTENTS

STATISTICS AND DATA ANALYTICS

FOR HEALTH DATA MANAGEMENT

UNDERSTANDING THE BASICS OF STATISTICS AND DATA ANALYTICS

CHAPTER 1

INTRODUCTION TO STATISTICAL TERMS AND CONCEPTS IN HEALTH DATA MANAGEMENT

CHAPTER OUTLINE

NUMBERS AT WORK
    Definitions and Significance
        Collection of Data
        Analysis of the Data
        Interpretation of the Data
        Presentation of Data

Data and Data Analytics
    Data
    Information
    Knowledge
    Business Intelligence
Uses and Users of Health Care
    Data

TYPES OF STATISTICS
HEALTH CARE DATA
    CLASSIFICATIONS
    Qualitative Data
    Quantitative Data
OBTAINING AND COMPARING
    HEALTH CARE DATA
REVIEW QUESTIONS

KEY TERMS

benchmarking
business intelligence
continuous data
data
data analytics
data set
descriptive statistics
inferential statistics

information
interval level data
knowledge
nominal level data
ordinal level data
population
primary data
qualitative data

quantitative data
ratio level data
sample
secondary data
statistics
value
variable

LEARNING OBJECTIVES

At the conclusion of this chapter, you should be able to:
1. Explain the importance of statistics and data analytics in health care.
2. Identify the users and uses of health care data.
3. Explain the difference between descriptive and inferential statistics.
4. Classify the levels of data measurement.
5. Differentiate populations and samples.
6. Distinguish common health care data sets and databases.

NUMBERS AT WORK

Every day on the news, in articles on the Internet, and from our books and instructors in the classroom, we read and hear about *numbers*. Maybe you have heard a commercial or a news reporter making a claim beginning with, "*Studies show…*"

- Four out of five dentists recommend brushing with Minty Sparkles toothpaste.
- Candidate X leads Candidate Y by 13 points in the latest poll.
- Fifty percent of the United States population now lives in cities.

These are all examples of numbers that have been put to work. A toothpaste marketer hopes that a strong recommendation for her brand might get you to try their product. When Candidate X reads the polling results, the numbers will tell her that she has been running a good campaign, and when Candidate Y finds out that he is 13 points behind his opponent, he will likely change his approach. A company might consider the percentage of people living in urban areas when choosing when or where to expand its business. In each case, the numbers are telling us about the way things are so that we know what to do next.

Contemporary health care is a business, too, and like most businesses, health care is driven by numbers. Most people have heard about the high costs of treatment, for example, or the increasing percentage of visits to emergency rooms. We might read about a facility with questionable death rates, desirable careers with attractive salaries, and hospitals forced to close because of low occupancy rates. These are all numbers derived from health care data—numbers that help us understand how health care is working, what we can expect, and how we can improve.

BRIEF CASE

USING WHAT YOU KNOW

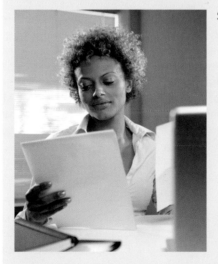

Sasha has always been described as a caring, organized, talented problem solver. When she graduated from high school, she looked forward to a career in health care, but was torn between direct patient care and administrative work. Fascinated with medicine, she decided to use her strengths to work with information collected in health care settings. Currently she works as a health care analyst with Diamonte Health, a hospital system that includes several hospitals and physician practices. Her days involve analyzing its enormous volume of data to monitor care, build reports, and measure progress toward those goals. One of her first courses was a statistics course, and she looks back at the concepts covered in the course as she goes through her day.

Definitions and Significance

So what are statistics and data analytics, and how do they apply to health care? Let us take a moment to define some terms. *Health care* is the discipline of diagnosing, preventing, and treating diseases and disorders. This definition also includes the organizational structure necessary to provide this care. **Statistics** is the scientific application of mathematical principles to the collection, analysis, interpretation, and presentation of numerical data. Essentially, statistics is a branch of mathematics that helps us gather and understand numerical data. When we put these two together, we get *health care statistics*, the application of

Statistics The scientific application of mathematical principles to the collection, analysis, interpretation, and presentation of numerical data.

mathematical principles to the *collection, analysis, interpretation*, and *presentation* of numerical data, to prevent and treat diseases and disorders. HIM professionals perform these tasks every day to facilitate patient care. Let us examine each of these functions more closely.

Collection of Data

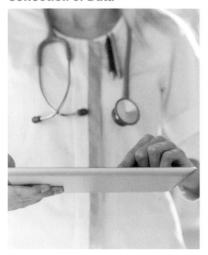

In hospitals, physician offices, and other health care provider settings the data consist largely of the administrative, financial, and clinical data collected by the facility or clinicians. The data—all those names, addresses, diagnoses, procedures, test results—are constantly being collected at the point of care and stored by providers of health care, insurance companies, and government agencies. Collection can also be done manually from medical charts (this is called *abstracting*) or digitally from electronic health records (EHRs) or management information systems. These data are organized into registries or indexes to make it easy to use. For example, a list of patient discharges sorted by the physician who treated them is called a *physician index*. A list of procedures performed over a certain period of time is called a *procedure index*. For example, the number of deliveries by month can be accessed by an examination of the procedure index through the use of the appropriate procedures, identified using ICD-10 codes (Figure 1-1).

EHR Electronic health record.

Analysis of the Data

Once the data are collected, HIM professionals can use it to answer questions about what is going on in the hospital. Imagine that a hospital administrator passes by a mother and

Z38.00	Single liveborn, born in hospital, delivered without mention of caesarian section	
Month	**Principal diagnosis**	**Number of babies born**
Jan	Z38.00	24
Feb	Z38.00	27
Mar	Z38.00	30
Apr	Z38.00	31
May	Z38.00	27
Jun	Z38.00	26
Jul	Z38.00	50
Aug	Z38.00	60
Sep	Z38.00	112
Oct	Z38.00	90
Nov	Z38.00	37
Dec	Z38.00	38
Average		46

Figure 1-1 Procedure index.

her new baby on her way into work one morning. When she leaves that day, she again notices a young family with a new baby leaving the hospital. "Wow," she thinks, "there are a lot of babies being born here recently." But how many is "a lot?" If 24 babies were born at the hospital last month, is that number less than last month? Is it lower than usual? Is it less than average? Analysis involves an initial question or problem that needs to be answered, and the calculations performed to address the question. In this case, the question might be: *what is the average number of deliveries by month in the last year?*

Interpretation of the Data

As HIM professionals, we are increasingly likely to be called on to create information from data that have been collected. Interpretation is the explanation of the results of the analysis. A hospital administrator might ask Sasha, whom we met at the beginning of the chapter, to investigate the number of babies born by month and report on her findings. Looking at the data, Sasha reports that the average monthly deliveries were 46, with a range from 24 in January to a high of 112 in September.

Presentation of Data

Presentation is the organization of the data into a format that allows for an understanding of the findings. There are a number of presentation tools commonly used in statistical analysis, and the usual formats for presentation are tables, charts, and graphs. In Chapter 3, we will explore these presentation tools and their uses in detail. See Table 1-1 for a summary.

■ EXERCISE 1-1
Numbers at Work

1. What is the purpose of health care statistics?

2. Which of the following is a graphical display of data over time?

   a. Pie chart
   b. Line graph
   c. Histogram
   d. Table

○ **Data** Items, observations, or raw facts.

○ **Data analytics** The inspection and evaluation of groups of data using statistics to answer questions and develop conclusions.

Data and Data Analytics

Statistics starts with **data**, which are the items, observations, or raw facts used to describe a question under study. These are the individual items that are collected.

The inspection and evaluation of groups of data using statistics are called **data analytics**, and this is the science with which HIM professionals answer questions and develop conclusions. Data analytics can be viewed as a hierarchy of tasks that begin with raw data and their maintenance and culminate with the use of statistics to make decisions about a variety of questions. We can arrange these tasks into the shape of a pyramid (Figure 1-2).

Data

Examples of data items in health care are as varied as patient age, sex, marital status, and diagnosis. Figure 1-3 shows some of the types of data items that are regularly collected on patients. Because of the all-inclusive nature of health care data, it would also include the salaries of nurses, the cost of medical office space, the outcome of medical procedures, and the results of diagnostic testing. We can divide the types of data

TABLE 1-1

PRESENTATION TOOLS AND THEIR USES

PRESENTATION TOOL	CONSTRUCTION	PURPOSE	EXAMPLE
Table	Column and rows. Construction depends on the items being compared.	Used to compare characteristics of items. Note in this table that the items are listed in the first column and the two characteristics (construction and purpose) head the comparison columns.	
Bar graph	Bars are drawn to represent the frequency of items in the specified categories of a variable. One axis represents the category. The other axis represents the frequency.	Used to compare categories with each other, the same category in different time periods, or both.	
Line graph	The horizontal (x) axis represents the observation. The vertical (y) axis represents the value of the observation. A point is made that corresponds to each observation, and a line is drawn to connect the points.	Used to represent data over a period of time; information is plotted along the x and y axes.	
Pie chart	In a circle, the percentage of each category is represented by a wedge of the circle that corresponds to the percentage of the circle.	Used to compare categories with one another in relation to the whole group.	
Histogram	Like a bar graph, but the sides of the bars are touching. Horizontally, each bar represents a class interval. Vertically, the height of the bar represents the frequency of the class interval.	Used to illustrate a frequency distribution.	

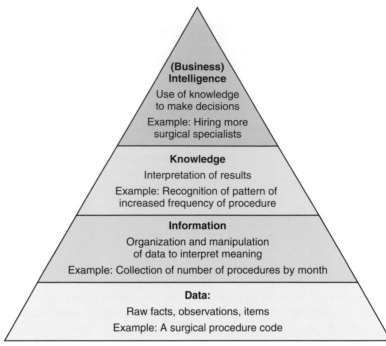

Figure 1-2 Data pyramid.

collected into several categories: departmental data, financial data, clinical data, and administrative (demographic and socioeconomic) data, and subsequent chapters will address each of these categories separately.

Information

The ultimate goal of health care statistics is to organize the data into a format that can be used to make decisions. Once we find the needed data, they must be organized to create **information**. The terms data and information are often used synonymously, but they are not the same. Data are the units of observation, and information is data that we have organized to have context and meaning. Health care information includes the calculations of median patient age, frequency of procedures, and average length of stay. The presentation of these results, whether that means formatting the data into tables and charts or presenting it in a PowerPoint presentation, is also a form of information.

> ⬤ **Information** Data that have been organized to give it context and meaning.

Knowledge

As information is created, patterns can be observed. Repetition of similar patterns over time or in multiple instances builds confidence in the user that the sequence of events demonstrated in the pattern is predictable. For example, assume a patient with steadily increasing blood pressure is given a drug that dilates blood vessels. The patient takes the drug, and then the blood pressure subsides to within normal limits. Observing this pattern—high blood pressure, take drug, blood pressure goes down—leads a pharmaceutical company to conclude that the drug lowers blood pressure. In this example, the information becomes **knowledge**, the conclusion arrived at by using information to determine a truth.

> ⬤ **Knowledge** Is the conclusion arrived at by using information to determine a truth.

> ⬤ **Business intelligence** Is the application of knowledge to make decisions.

Business Intelligence

Finally, **business intelligence** is the top of the pyramid and the final use of the collection, analysis, interpretation, and presentation of data. Once the data have been organized and analyzed, researchers and administrators can use the findings to make decisions regarding critical areas of concern; whether they are of a clinical or an administrative nature.

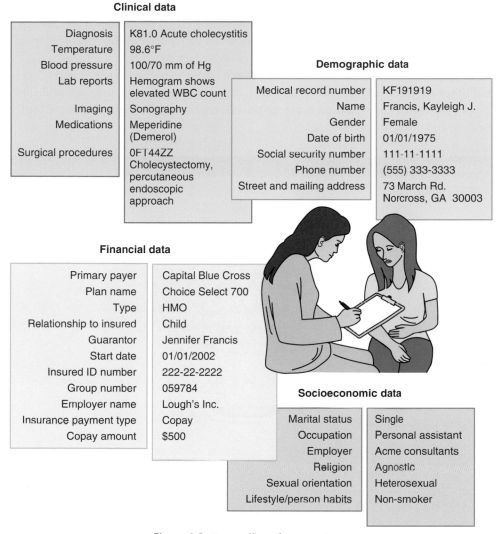

Clinical data

Diagnosis	K81.0 Acute cholecystitis
Temperature	98.6°F
Blood pressure	100/70 mm of Hg
Lab reports	Hemogram shows elevated WBC count
Imaging	Sonography
Medications	Meperidine (Demerol)
Surgical procedures	0FT44ZZ Cholecystectomy, percutaneous endoscopic approach

Demographic data

Medical record number	KF191919
Name	Francis, Kayleigh J.
Gender	Female
Date of birth	01/01/1975
Social security number	111-11-1111
Phone number	(555) 333-3333
Street and mailing address	73 March Rd. Norcross, GA 30003

Financial data

Primary payer	Capital Blue Cross
Plan name	Choice Select 700
Type	HMO
Relationship to insured	Child
Guarantor	Jennifer Francis
Start date	01/01/2002
Insured ID number	222-22-2222
Group number	059784
Employer name	Lough's Inc.
Insurance payment type	Copay
Copay amount	$500

Socioeconomic data

Marital status	Single
Occupation	Personal assistant
Employer	Acme consultants
Religion	Agnostic
Sexual orientation	Heterosexual
Lifestyle/person habits	Non-smoker

Figure 1-3 Data collected on a patient.

Uses and Users of Health Care Data

Why do health care professionals collect all these data? The primary purpose of recording data is communication, which is necessary to deliver patient care. The most obvious is use by clinicians for direct patient care involving diagnosis and treatment. Physicians must document their orders for patient care, and nurses document the patient's progress, vital signs, and medications they administered.

An admissions staff member records the patient's health insurance data to communicate with the payer (i.e., to be paid for services rendered to the patient). A nurse scans a patient's wristband so that everyone knows the right patient received the right medication (Figure 1-4). Observations about the patient's medical condition are recorded by one party (e.g., a nurse) for the benefit of another party (e.g., a physician). Each service rendered to a patient is captured or collected, partly for payment purposes, but also to help the provider know what staff resources have been used and what supplies need to be restocked. We call this kind of data collected or generated by clinicians when treating a patient **primary data**, the original, firsthand account of the patient's treatment.

In addition, managers use data for planning, organizing, controlling, directing, and staffing health care facilities. Payers (insurance companies) use patient data to determine allowable reimbursement; researchers also use patient data, but to test the possibility of improved diagnostic techniques and treatments. These data users probably would not look at individual patient records. Instead, certain data are selected and

Primary data In health care, items that are obtained directly from the patient record and which specifically identify that patient.

○ **Secondary data** Summarized or abstracted items that may or may not be patient identifiable.

reported from individual patient records in a process called abstracting, and then organized separately in a list or index. The type of data is called **secondary data**, and they come from sources other than the original recorder or reporter of the data. The procedure index in Figure 1-1 is a good example of secondary data.

In general, users of health data can be divided into internal and external users. Internal users are those within the facilities including the departments, services, and caregivers; whereas the external users are the payers, regulating (licensing and accrediting) bodies, and government agencies.

BRIEF CASE

USING QUALITY DATA

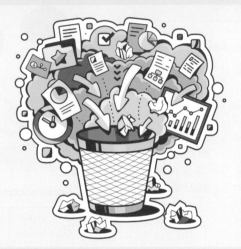

Professionals who work with health care data have a responsibility to maintain clean and accurate data. One of Sasha's tasks is maintenance of the master patient index. As part of her job, she runs a monthly report to check for duplications, errors, and missing information. Over her desk she has a poster that reminds her of the importance of data quality. She is well aware that any work she does with the data is only as good as the quality of the data itself.

■ EXERCISE 1-2

Uses and Users of Health Care Data

1. Which of the following is an example of primary data collection?

   a. An HIM professional abstracts data from patient records into a database.
   b. A nurse records a patient's blood pressure during an office visit.
   c. A hospital administrator generates a report of the number of tonsillectomies performed last year.
   d. A researcher examines reports of gunshot wounds from trauma centers.

2. You use the physician index to find out how many patient discharges Dr. Daulis had last month. This is a use of _____ data.

TYPES OF STATISTICS

○ **Descriptive statistics** The analytical activities and calculations performed to explain what is or what was.

There are two main types of statistics: *descriptive* and *inferential*. **Descriptive statistics**, which will probably fill the majority of one's time at a health care facility, is the discipline

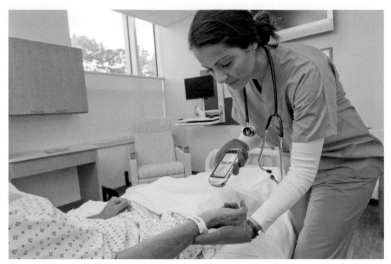

Figure 1-4 Zebra scanning technology is used to help improve patient identification and safety. (Courtesy Zebra Technologies Corporation, Lincolnshire, IL).

of collecting, describing, interpreting, and presenting data. The data that are studied are called a **population** because it is *all* of the patients, salaries, doctors, etc., that are being examined for their characteristics.

In contrast, **inferential statistics** is the study of using mathematical models to *predict* future events and to draw conclusions about a sample of a population. This type of statistics is useful not only when you want to be able to numerically describe a particular characteristic but also when you want to be able to conclude (with some certainty) that those characteristics extend to similar future groups. A **sample** is a subset of the population that has been selected using a particular sampling method. In short, descriptive statistics describes the data that are either in the past or present of a population, while inferential statistics helps make an intelligent guess about what the data would be in the future from a sample.

For example, descriptive statistics answers questions about how many patients visited the emergency room last year; how long patients stayed in the hospital with a particular diagnosis for the month of August; what was the average total cholesterol level of patients with type II diabetes this year to date; which insurance carrier had the highest accounts receivable balance last week; and which zip code was connected to the greatest number of patients this year.

On the other hand, inferential statistics answers questions about how many patients can we expect in the emergency room *next year*; which physician practice can be expected to bring in the highest revenue *next year*; what *will be* the probable survival of a patient with stage IV inflammatory breast cancer; or how likely is it that patients with surgical complications *will require* readmission within 7 days of discharge? In this textbook, we will explore descriptive statistics in Unit 2 and introduce inferential statistics in Unit 3.

○ A population Is a complete group of all of the items that are under study.

○ Inferential statistics The study of using mathematical models to *predict* future events.

○ A sample Is a subset of the population that has been selected using a particular sampling method.

TAKE AWAY ●·········

Descriptive statistics *describes*, while inferential statistics *predicts*. Descriptive statistics measures a complete population, while inferential statistics measures a sample of a population.

EXERCISE 1-3

1. Measles is very rare in the United States. A group of researchers was able to collect demographic and clinical data from all 55 reported cases. These researchers used a:

   a. Sample
   b. Population

○ **Variable** An item or characteristic that is measured or counted.

○ **Value** The count or measurement of the observation.

HEALTH CARE DATA CLASSIFICATIONS

Our health care data can be characterized in a variety of ways. One set of important definitions to understand and differentiate is that of **variables** and **values**. Any item or characteristic that we may want to measure or count (the number of patients, an A1c level, patient's weight, reimbursement) is called a *variable*. The individual observations of the variables being measured (18 patients, a 5.9% A1c, 134 pounds, $4328) are called *values*. For students, an example of a common variable is a test grade. A value would be the grade received for one particular test.

Variables can be categorized as independent or dependent. Independent variables are the ones that are chosen and varied by the researcher. They are often described as the cause of whatever response is measured. The response, or effect, is measured in what is called the dependent variable. To follow the student example using grades, we could measure:

- number of hours spent studying for an exam (independent)/grade received (dependent)
- number of cups of coffee consumed within 24 hours of an exam (independent)/exam grade (dependent)
- number of friends taking the same exam (independent)/exam grade (dependent).

Examples from health care for independent/dependent pairs would be:
- diagnosis (independent)/mortality rate (dependent)
- weeks of gestation (independent)/weight in grams (dependent)
- month (independent)/patient census (dependent)

A good way to test if you have the independent and dependent values sorted out correctly is to flip them around and see if the opposite scenario could make sense. While the number of cups of coffee consumed before an exam could influence an exam grade, it is impossible for the exam grade to influence the number of cups of coffee consumed before that exam.

In the process of organizing multitudes of health care data, the data that are collected for the values that measure our variables can be divided into two broad categories: those that represent groups of categories (qualitative) and those that are expressed as numbers (quantitative). Figure 1-5 shows how data are categorized.

TAKE AWAY ●·········

Independent variables are the suspected cause, while dependent variables are the presumed effect.

Stat Tip ···

Knowing the difference between qualitative and quantitative data is important because as you gain an understanding of the types of statistics that can be used, you will need to choose statistical formulas based on the level of data measurement that has been collected. Inferential statistics uses tests that have the analyst choose between *parametric* tests (those that are used in "normal" populations and use mostly interval and ratio data) and *nonparametric* tests (those that can be used to analyze nonnormal populations and are most often nominal and ordinal data). The normal and nonnormal categorizations have to do with concepts that will be covered in Unit 3. For now, pay attention to the levels of data measurement and be able to recognize and sort them into their respective categories.

○ **Qualitative data** Observations without a numerical value that can be sorted or counted into categories.

TAKE AWAY ●··········

Qualitative data can be counted or sorted but not added together.

Qualitative Data

Qualitative data can be sorted into categories but cannot be measured. Such data have no real numerical value. Examples of qualitative data in health care are marital status, diagnosis, insurance carrier, nursing unit, grades of sprains (mild, moderate, severe), and Likert scales in patient satisfaction surveys (least to most satisfied). These types of data are recognized for being able to be classified into a specific category and can be counted for the totals in each category.

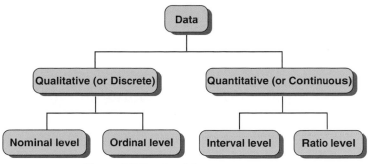

Figure 1-5 Levels of data measurement.

Qualitative data can be subdivided into two levels of measurement. **Nominal level data** are descriptive and have no logical order, like a listing of insurance carriers. A patient's personal identifier (medical record number), gender, race, and ethnicity are all nominal data. But even though nominal data have no numerical value, the data can still be counted. This means that we can add the number of observations of such data and perform calculations on the sum. Look at Figure 1-6. Can you see how you could sort these examples into their respective categories and that the totals in each category could be reported? But you cannot really "measure" marital status. That is, there is no arithmetic or sequential relationship between the observations. The categories are married, single, divorced, or widowed, not "how much of each." You cannot, for instance, be 50% widowed. And there is no value relationship: one is not more or better than the other.

Ordinal level data are descriptive too, but it also has an inherent natural order. Examples include a patient satisfaction survey ranging from least to most satisfied, or grades of sprains. However, there is still no arithmetic relationship among the observations: one "very satisfied" plus one "neutral" does not equal one "very satisfied."

Nominal level data A type of qualitative data without a mathematical relationship or order among observations.

Ordinal level data A type of nominal data in which the observations have an ordered value.

TAKE AWAY

Two types of qualitative data are nominal and ordinal data.

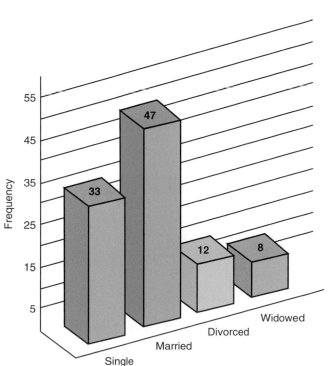

Figure 1-6 Since marital status is a type of nominal data, it can be counted but not measured.

You may hear the term *discrete data*. These data are those that are represented by totals for the categories and are represented by whole numbers (47 married patients, 8 widowed, 33 single, and 12 divorced). Qualitative data are discrete data.

Stat Tip ··

Not all texts use the term "qualitative" to refer to this type of data. Synonyms for qualitative data are dichotomous, binary, categorical, and discrete data.

○ **Quantitative data** Numeric data.

○ **Interval level data** A type of quantitative data without a natural zero, in which the values may be added or subtracted but multiplying and dividing them have no meaning.

○ **Ratio level data** A type of quantitative data with a meaningful, natural zero in its order.

○ **Continuous data** Data on a scale in which numbers have values in between the whole numbers.

TAKE AWAY ●··········

Quantitative data (interval and ratio data) have numerical value and can have some arithmetic relationships; however, only ratio data have a true zero value, enabling all mathematical functions.

Quantitative Data

Quantitative data can be measured numerically (by age, weight, height, time, dollars, etc.), and these data may be used for calculations to further describe their group (patients, hours per week, or salaries). As a matter of fact, a major distinguishing feature between quantitative and qualitative data is that while qualitative data are represented by categories, quantitative data are numerical. Again, there are two categories of qualitative data.

Interval level data have a logical order or ranking, and the intervals are meaningful, but the concept of a natural zero is missing. A temperature scale is a kind of interval level data: if it is 0 °C outside, it does not mean that there is no temperature at all. Because of that, any ratios developed have no meaning. Normal body temperature is 37 °C, and 40 °C is 3 °C higher, but is not 108% hotter than normal body temperature. We are able to add and subtract degrees on the scale, but multiplying and dividing them has no meaning.

On the other hand, **ratio level data** have a logical order or ranking, meaningful, consistent intervals, and include a zero in its order. The observation may be multiplied or divided to produce meaningful results. For example, a patient who weighs 100 kg is twice as heavy as one who weighs 50 kg. Let us look at some other examples.

Ratio level data in health care include patient ages, weights, lengths of stay, salaries, and billing charges. **Continuous data** are represented by numbers that have values in between the whole numbers (temperatures: 37.4, 98.6; weights; time; and salaries: $32,450.81, $49,341.28). Although we generally express age as a number of days, months, or years, age is really continuous data, in that a person could be 45.937 years old. Since we start the age clock at birth, age had an absolute zero (not born). Therefore, someone who is 30 years old is twice as old as someone who is 15 years old. Age is an important data element in analyzing health care data because we often look at events, such as procedures and the onset of illnesses, in terms of when they occurred in the patient's life.

EXERCISE 1-4

Health Care Data Classifications

	A	B	C	D	E	F	G
1	Hospital name	Discharges	Total days	ADC	Mean LOS	Mean charge per discharge	Case-mix adjusted charge per discharge
2	Auburn Regional Medical Center	7110	27,701	75.89	3.90	29,743.28	33,781.33
3	Central Washington Hospital	10,157	34,085	93.38	3.36	22,337.24	21,253.45
4	Deaconess Hospital	10,631	49,164	134.70	4.62	34,029.19	31,557.78
5	Evergreen Hospital Medical Center	20,252	63,998	175.34	3.16	22,194.44	28,254.54
6	Grays Harbor Community Hospital	5870	20,156	55.22	3.43	21,161.13	26,009.65
7	Harborview Medical Center	17,838	109,047	298.76	6.11	56,008.23	35,351.05
8	Harrison Memorial Hospital	16,028	60,407	165.50	3.77	36,817.31	36,323.82

Look at the spreadsheet above to answer the following questions.

EXERCISE 1-4
Health Care Data Classifications—cont'd

1. True or false: there are no nominal level data listed in the spreadsheet.

   a. True
   b. False

2. The values in the "Discharges" category are:

   a. Qualitative data
   b. Rounded up
   c. Continuous data
   d. Ratio level data

3. The values in the "Mean Charge per Discharge" column are expressed in dollars. This is a type of:

   a. Qualitative data
   b. Interval level data
   c. Continuous data
   d. Nominal data

BRIEF CASE

RUNNING THE NUMBERS

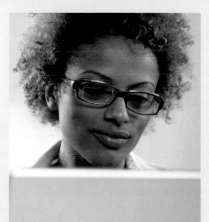

● **MA** Medical assistant.

One of the practice managers in Sasha's health system has insisted that the other practices have more medical assistants (MAs) per patient than his practice and that they are paid a higher average salary. Sasha has been asked to report on the salaries of MAs employed by each of the seven physician practice groups. The administrator has asked Sasha to "run the numbers" and check the staffing and salaries at each of the practices.

1. Measuring the number of MAs by physician practice group is what level of data?
   a. Nominal
   b. Ordinal
   c. Ratio
   d. Interval

2. Measuring the MA salaries is what level of data?
   a. Nominal
   b. Ordinal
   c. Ratio
   d. Interval

OBTAINING AND COMPARING HEALTH CARE DATA

Statistical analysis is only one part of a researcher's task. Findings often benefit from a comparison to data that have already been collected and to other established standards. The secondary data sources that were noted earlier (disease and procedure indices, along

TJC The Joint Commision.

Benchmarking Is the process of comparing one's results to standards or references.

HAI Hospital-acquired infection.

Data set A standard group of elements collected so that they can be compared with similar data.

SNF Skilled nursing facility.

UHDDS Uniform Hospital Discharge Data Set.

MDS Minimum Data Set.

UACDS Uniform Ambulatory Care Data Set.

with cancer and trauma registries), in addition to public and private standards, provide data that can be used to compare results. For example, the Joint Commission (TJC) had established standards of care for treating myocardial infarctions. These standards included giving patients aspirin on admission and again at discharge. Hospitals measured their success on these two measures and compared themselves against national and local results.

Benchmarking is the process of comparing one's results to standards or references. To do that, a data analyst must be aware of the types of data that are collected and the form(s) in which they appear. Part of data maintenance is being sure that those forms are accurate with all of the digits/characters and decimal points in the correct places. ICD-10-CM/PCS codes have different numbers of characters and digits. Diagnosis coding under this system uses three to seven alpha and numeric characters that include a decimal point after the first three characters. The procedure coding uses seven alpha/numeric characters without a decimal point.

Medicare's Hospital Compare Website (http://www.medicare.gov/hospitalcompare/) allows the public to evaluate up to three hospitals at a time in nationally reported measures such as readmission rates, hospital-acquired infections (HAI), and patient satisfactions. The results are reported as "better, worse, or no different" and percentages of patients' agreement with a number of different survey questions. Clinicians routinely compare test results to a range of normal/abnormal results.

A **data set** is a standard group of elements collected so that they can be compared with similar data, collected either in a different time or from a different facility. Without a standardized, defined data set, comparison or benchmarking is difficult. Imagine that one skilled nursing facility (SNF) has been collecting data on the primary occupation of its new residents since it opened 30 years ago. In that time, a total of 10 patients under their care were diagnosed with mesothelioma, a form of cancer usually caused by asbestos exposure. Almost all of these patients worked at the local packaging plant. A neighboring SNF counts 15 cases of mesothelioma over this time period, but it has only collected data on its patients' occupation for the past 3 years. Without a means of comparing their cases to the incidence of mesothelioma in the general population, along with a defined data set that collects the information, it is impossible to determine whether the second SNF's incidence of mesothelioma is connected to the packaging plant.

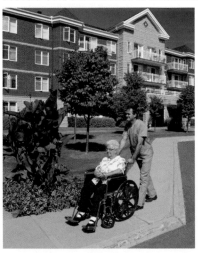

For most types of health care delivery, a minimum set of data must be collected and reported for each patient. Hospitals, for example, are required to collect certain information from all their inpatients, including the patient's name, the dates the patient was admitted to and discharged from the facility, diagnoses given, and procedures performed, among other things. This is called the Uniform Hospital Discharge Data Set (UHDDS); a summary of its elements are shown in Box 1-1. Some other examples of data sets include the Minimum Data Set (MDS) for nursing home facilities and the Uniform Ambulatory Care Data Set (UACDS) collected by outpatient settings, such as clinics and physician's offices.

TAKE AWAY ● •

Most types of health care delivery require a minimum set of data collected and reported for each patient.

Once data sets are collected, data analysts can avail themselves of several national databases to compare their results. A summary of a few of the data sources that may be used to benchmark data is displayed in Table 1-2.

BRIEF CASE

CHECKING THE CODES

Sasha runs a report of procedures performed by one of the physicians in the last month. As she looks over the results before giving it to the physician, she sees that 10 of the surgeries are recorded with one character and two digits. Why is this a concern?

BOX 1-1   UNIFORM HOSPITAL DISCHARGE DATA SET (UHDDS) SUMMARY OF DATA ELEMENTS

- Personal/unique identifier
- Date of birth
- Gender
- Race and ethnicity
- Residence
- Health care facility identification number
- Admission date
- Type of admission
- Discharge date
- Attending physician's identification number
- Surgeon's identification number
- Principal diagnosis
- Other diagnoses
- Qualifier for other diagnoses
- External cause of injury
- Birth weight of neonate
- Significant procedures and dates of procedures
- Disposition of the patient at discharge
- Expected source of payment
- Total charges

▪ EXERCISE 1-5

▪ Obtaining and Comparing Health Care Data

1. You need to prepare a report on the birth weights of newborns at your hospital for each quarter of the year. Where do you think you could get these data?

   a. DEEDS
   b. HEDIS
   c. ORYX
   d. UHDDS

2. What is the name of the data set collected by Medicare- and Medicaid-certified nursing homes?

   a. Healthcare Effectiveness Data and Information Set (HEDIS)
   b. Minimum Data Set (MDS)
   c. Outcome and Assessment Information Set (OASIS)
   d. Uniform Ambulatory Care Data Set (UACDS)

TABLE 1-2

DATABASES AND DATA SETS USED FOR BENCHMARKING

DATABASES AND DATA SETS	MAINTAINED BY	TYPES OF DATA	WEBSITE ADDRESS
Data Elements for Emergency Department Systems (DEEDS)	US Government	A set of data elements to provide uniformity in collection of emergency department data.	http://www.cdc.gov/ncipc/pub-res/pdf/deeds.pdf
Healthcare Effectiveness Data and Information Set (HEDIS)	NCQA	HEDIS is a tool used to measure performance on important dimensions of care and service in the majority of health plans.	http://www.ncqa.org/HEDISQualityMeasurement.aspx
Minimum Data Set (MDS)	US Government	The Minimum Data Set (MDS) is part of a nationally mandated process for clinical assessment of all residents in Medicare- or Medicaid-certified nursing homes.	http://www.cms.gov/Research-Statistics-Data-and-Systems/Computer-Data-and-Systems/MDSPubQIandResRep/index.html?redirect=/MDSPubQIandResRep/
Outcome and Assessment Information Set (OASIS)	US Government	This data set is for use in home health agencies (HHAs), state agencies, software vendors, professional associations, and other Federal agencies in implementing and maintaining OASIS. The home health agencies that desire Medicare certification are required to meet Medicare's Conditions of Participation. Part of the Conditions is compliance with the collection and transmission of OASIS data elements.	http://www.cms.gov/Medicare/Quality-Initiatives-Patient-Assessment-Instruments/OASIS/index.html
ORYX* for Hospitals (National Hospital Quality Measures)	The Joint Commission	ORYX* is the Joint Commission's performance measurement and improvement initiative, which integrates outcomes and other performance measure data into the accreditation process. The data from ORYX are reported on the Joint Commission website at Quality Check*, www.qualitycheck.org, allowing public comparisons of hospital performance at both state and national levels.	http://www.jointcommission.org/facts_about_oryx_for_hospitals/
Uniform Ambulatory Care Data Set (UACDS)	National Uniform Claim Committee	A set of data elements to provide uniformity in outpatient settings, collected on a form called the CMS-1500.	http://www.nucc.org/
Uniform Hospital Discharge Data Set (UHDDS)	National Uniform Billing Committee (NUBC)	A set of data elements to provide uniformity in hospital inpatient data, collected on a form called the UB-04.	http://www.nubc.org/
National Cancer Database (NCDB)	American College of Surgeons, the Commission on Cancer, and American Cancer Society	A nationwide oncology outcomes database for more than 1500 Commission-accredited cancer programs in the United States and Puerto Rico.	http://www.facs.org/cancer/ncdb/

1. What types of data items are collected in health care?

2. Tia is abstracting medical records to report on the use of completion of the free text fields. She is using which type of data?

   a. Primary
   b. Secondary

3. Veronica is asked to report the age, sex, and type of insurance for patients who had gastric bypass surgery last year. She would be using which type of statistics to calculate a response?

   a. Descriptive
   b. Inferential

4. Sex and race are examples of which type of data?

   a. Nominal
   b. Ordinal
   c. Ratio
   d. Interval

5. For a class project, you ask 100 people on campus how many hours they slept the night before. Your study is based on a:

   a. Population
   b. Sample

6. How are data sets used in health care?

BASIC MATH CONCEPTS, CENTRAL TENDENCY, AND DISPERSION

CHAPTER OUTLINE

KEY TERMS

class
cumulative frequency
decimal
dispersion
fraction
frequency
frequency distribution
mean

median
mode
percentage
proportion
quartiles
quotient
range
rate

ratio
relative frequency
rounding
standard deviation
variance
volume

LEARNING OBJECTIVES

At the conclusion of this chapter, you should be able to:

1. Perform calculations with fractions, decimals, and percentages.
2. Understand the function of rates, ratios, and proportions in health care statistics.
3. Explain why frequencies and frequency distributions are useful to data analysts.

4. Identify the most useful measure of central tendency for a given set of data.
5. Calculate the variance and standard deviation from a frequency distribution.

For some of you, this chapter may be a review that allows you to become reacquainted with concepts learned in an earlier academic setting. For others, this may be a necessary kick-start to the math required to carry out calculations used in health statistics and analytics. If you feel that you are solid on a concept, go ahead and try the exercises for that section. If you find that you are getting them right, by all means, go ahead to the next section. If not, there is no shame in taking the time to brush up on the areas that you may not have used for many years. Remember that the phrase "if you do not use it, you lose it" applies to math concepts and everything else in life.

Let us start by looking at some mathematical concepts that you encountered in school a long time ago.

Stat Tip ··

Medicine, like many sciences, uses the metric system to measure weights, lengths, and fluid volumes. Refer to the inside back cover of this text for a guide to converting metric and standard units.

BRIEF CASE

UNDERSTANDING THE POPULATION

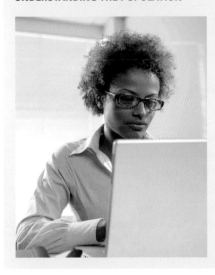

In the administration of any health care facility, the size and scope of the patient population help determine the resources needed to deliver care, like staffing and technology. Part of Sasha's job is to get a sense of the kinds of cases the hospital is treating, and the length of time it takes to treat those cases. To do this, she needs to look at some patient data and calculate the numbers of patients treated.

FRACTIONS, DECIMALS, AND PERCENTAGES

Fractions, decimals, and percentages are different ways of expressing the same values. Throughout your experience in health care, you will need to use these numbers to communicate your findings. Although these concepts are all related, they each often appear separately, and you will need to be able to use, calculate, and convert them to their related forms.

Fractions

Fractions are numbers that are expressed as parts of a whole. While we may not always recognize the use of fractions, they are common in our everyday lives. For example, every Friday night you might order a large pepperoni pizza. The pizza arrives already cut into eight pieces. On a normal Friday night, your very hungry roommate eats at

○ **Fractions** Numbers that are expressed as parts of a whole.

least five pieces of that whole pizza pie. If this were expressed as a fraction, we could say that he ate 5/8's of the pizza. The top number (his five pieces, called the numerator) is the parts of the whole that we measured, and the bottom number (8, called the denominator) is the total (whole) number of pieces.

Other examples include baking (you use a ¾ cup of brown sugar in your chocolate chip recipe); time (it takes you a half of an hour to walk my dog); parking (it costs a quarter to buy 12 minutes on a parking meter in the city); shopping (you get 1/3 off when using a coupon from the newspaper); and snow accumulation (we just got 13½ inches of snow). Can you think of some other examples? Note that each time, the numerator on the top is the number of parts, while the denominator on the bottom is the total number of parts that the piece is divided into. When the numerator and the denominator are the same, the fraction is equal to 1. For example, 4/4 = 1, 70/70 = 1, 14/14 = 1. If your roommate was really hungry and he ate 8/8 slices of pizza, then he ate one whole pie.

Simple fractions are those that are less a whole number (3/4, 6/7, 9/10), while compound fractions (also called a mixed number fractions) are those that represent numbers greater than one (1½, 3¾, 56¼). Compound fractions can also be expressed with a numerator that is larger than the denominator. These are sometimes called *improper* or *top-heavy* fractions. For example,

$$\frac{3}{2} \text{ is the same amount as } 1\frac{1}{2}$$

$$\frac{15}{4} \text{ is the same amount as } 3\frac{3}{4}$$

$$\text{and } \frac{225}{4} \text{ is the same amount as } 56\frac{1}{4}$$

You can convert an improper fraction to a mixed number fraction by dividing the numerator by the denominator to the nearest whole number and showing the amount left over (i.e., the amount less than one) as a fraction. In the second example above, we ask, how many 4s can fit into 15 without going over 15? Two 4s would be 8 (2×4), three 4s would be 12 (3×4), and four 4s would be 16 (4×4). Sixteen is too many, so we know we can fit 3 wholes of this fraction into 15. That leaves ¾ left over. The mixed number fraction ¹⁵⁄₄ is the same thing as saying 3¾.

We convert mixed number fractions to improper fractions by reversing the process. Multiply the denominator (in this example, 4) by the whole number (3) to get 12. Then add the remaining fraction (¾) to get 15/4. Figure 2-1 shows how both of these operations work.

Stat Tip ···

Did you know that the word fraction is derived from the Latin word *fractus* meaning broken? Fractures are broken bones, while fractions are numbers that are broken into parts.

● **ICU** Intensive care unit.

What are some examples of fractions in health care? We can use them any time we are working with parts of a whole. If there are 10 beds in the intensive care unit (ICU), and seven are filled, our fraction is 7/10. If we had 1000 discharges last year, and 13 of those patients had hospital-acquired pneumonia (meaning they contracted the disease while they were in the hospital), then the fractional representation is 13/1000.

¾ goes into ¹⁵⁄₄ 3 times with ¾ left over,

$$\frac{15}{4} = \left(\frac{4}{4}\right) + \left(\frac{4}{4}\right) + \left(\frac{4}{4}\right) + \frac{3}{4}$$

$$= 1 + 1 + 1 + \frac{3}{4}$$

$$= 3\frac{3}{4}$$

A

$$\begin{array}{c}12 \\ \| \\ 3\,\frac{3}{4}\end{array}$$
×

Step 1: Multiply the denominator (4) by the whole number (3)
$4 \times 3 = 12$

$$\begin{array}{c}12 + \\ 3\,\frac{3}{4}\end{array} = 15$$

Step 2: Add the numerator (3) to the sum of the denominator and whole number (12)
$12 + 3 = 15$ This is the new numerator (15)

$$3\,\frac{3}{4} \longrightarrow \frac{15}{4}$$

Step 3: Keep the same denominator (4)

Answer: $3\,\frac{3}{4} = \frac{15}{4}$

B

Figure 2-1 A, Converting an improper fraction to a mixed number fraction. **B,** converting a mixed number fraction to an improper fraction.

Frequently, we reduce fractions to make them easier to understand and to work with. If 10 of the 20 cribs in the nursery are full, we probably would not say the nursery is 10/20 (ten-twentieths) full. We would reduce the fraction to ½, and we would say that it is half-full. This works because of one of the neat things you can do with fractions: when you multiply or divide the numerator and the denominator by the same number (called a factor), it does not change the value of the fraction. For instance, consider the following:

$$\frac{10}{20} \div 10 = \frac{10 \div 10}{20 \div 10} = \frac{1}{2}$$

$$\frac{15}{20} \div 5 = \frac{15 \div 5}{20 \div 5} = \frac{3}{4}$$

$$\frac{16}{64} \div 8 = \frac{16 \div 8}{64 \div 8} = \frac{2}{8} \div 2 = \frac{2 \div 2}{8 \div 2} = \frac{1}{4}$$

Notice that in the last example, we did not reduce the fraction all the way to its simplest form the first time when we divided by 8. We could have skipped a step and divided 16/64 by 16 and still arrived at the same simplest fraction, ¼.

Multiplication works exactly the same way—we can multiply the fraction by whatever factor we want, as long as we do the same thing to both the numerator and the denominator.

$$\frac{2}{3} \times 10 = \frac{2 \times 10}{3 \times 10} = \frac{20}{30}$$

● MATH REVIEW

If my roommate eats 5/8 of the pizza and I eat 1/8, did we together eat 6/16?

No, we ate 6/8, or ¾ of the pie.

Changing fractions by multiplying and dividing is important because if we want to add or subtract them, the denominator has to be the same number. And we do not add the denominators, because that is just the total possible.

Let us say the medical-surgical (med-surg) unit on the second floor is 5/12 full, and the med-surg unit on the third floor is 1/12 full. Workers on the 3rd floor need to shut off the air conditioning for repairs, and the hospital decides to move (add) the patients from the 3rd floor to the 2nd floor. How many patients will be on the 2nd floor med-surg unit after the patients are moved? In this case, the addition is easy because the denominators are the same.

$$\frac{5}{12} + \frac{1}{12} = \frac{6}{12} = \frac{1}{2}$$

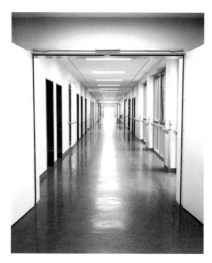

After the move, the unit on the 2nd floor will have 6 patients, and since there are 12 beds, it will be ½ full. But let us try adding fractions where the denominator is not the same. Say the 3rd floor was 1/3 full, and the 2nd floor is ½ full. Will there be enough room on the 2nd floor? (Note: 1/3 + ½ **does not** equal 2/5!)

To add (or subtract) fractions with different denominators, we must multiply the fractions by some factor first so that we are adding fractions with the same denominator. Remember, we can multiply or divide a fraction any way we want without changing its value, as long as we treat the denominator and the numerator the same.

$$\frac{1}{3} \times 2 = \frac{2}{6} \text{Patients from the 3rd floor}$$

$$\frac{1}{2} \times 3 = \frac{3}{6} \text{Patients on the 2nd floor}$$

$\frac{2}{6} + \frac{3}{6} = \frac{5}{6}$ Adding them together, the 2nd floor will be 5/6 full after the patients are moved.

EXERCISE 2-1
Fractions

1. Convert the following improper fractions to mixed number fractions:

    a. $\dfrac{12}{8}$

    b. $\dfrac{5}{2}$

    c. $\dfrac{144}{12}$

2. Convert the following mixed number fractions to improper fractions:

    a. $3\dfrac{3}{8}$

    b. $13\dfrac{1}{2}$

    c. $7\dfrac{5}{16}$

3. Reduce the fractions below to their simplest form.

    a. $\dfrac{2}{8}$

    b. $\dfrac{50}{100}$

    c. $\dfrac{75}{1000}$

    d. $\dfrac{12}{144}$

    e. $\dfrac{6}{36}$

4. Add or subtract the following fractions. Report your answers in simple fractions.

    a. $\dfrac{1}{8} + \dfrac{7}{12}$

    b. $\dfrac{7}{8} - \dfrac{1}{16}$

    c. $\dfrac{1}{2} - \dfrac{1}{5}$

    d. $\dfrac{2}{3} + 1\dfrac{1}{3}$

    e. $3\dfrac{5}{8} + 7\dfrac{3}{4}$

WORKING WITH FRACTIONS

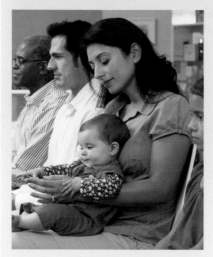

One of the clinics attached to the hospital system handles walk-ins and provides some urgent care services. Of the 120 patients seen last month, 10 were Asian-American, 35 were Latino or Hispanic, and 15 were African-American. Sasha wants to report these ethnicities in simple fractions.

Determine the fraction of the whole for each ethnic group and report your findings in simple fractions.

Asian-American:
Latino or Hispanic:
African-American:

Decimals

> **Decimal** A fraction with a denominator based on a power of 10.

Decimals are related to fractions in that they are numbers that are divided into units of 10. **Decimals** are actually fractions whose denominators are some power of 10 (10, 100, 1000, etc.) and are written as a decimal point followed by the numerator. For example, the fraction 1/10 (one-tenth) can be written as the decimal 0.1. $7^{64}/_{100}$ (seven and sixty-four one-hundredths) is expressed as 7.64 in decimal form. Again, these numbers, like fractions, are describing parts of a whole. The difference between fractions and decimals is not only in the way they look, but also in the concept of a whole. In decimals, the whole is always divisible by 10 (for example: 10, 100, 1000). The decimal point separates the whole from the parts (like the line between numerator and denominator), but in decimals, the whole numbers are to the left of the decimal point, while the parts are to the right. Figure 2-2 shows the numbers that each of the placeholders represents, along with its notation and the prefixes associated with each.

TAKE AWAY

Decimals, like fractions, describe parts of a whole.

Changing Fractions to Decimals

Sometimes, you will need to change a fraction into a decimal for performing a calculation. A great example is the sale coupon that gives you 1/3 off of your purchase. One of the t-shirts that would be perfect for my niece (and my budget) is priced at $36.00. If it

Place Value and Decimals													
Millions	Hundred thousands	Ten thousands	Thousands	Hundreds	Tens	Ones	Decimal point	Tenths	Hundredths	Thousandths	Ten-thousandths	Hundred-thousandths	Millionths
			4	8	2	9	.	1	7				

Figure 2-2 Decimal placeholders.

is 1/3 off, how much will I save? I might first think to divide the price into three's, then multiply by two. A third off would be the following:

$$\frac{36}{3} = 12 \times 2 = \$24. \text{ I saved } \$12.$$

But, you can also change the 1/3 into a decimal, then multiply it by the price to see how much you are going to save. Let us say a second, equally enticing t-shirt is 2/5 off and is priced at $39. $39 is not easily divisible by 5, so making that fraction (2/5) into a decimal might be easier. To convert, we just divide the numerator (which is 2) by the denominator (5) to get the **quotient.**

Quotient The result of division.

$$2 \div 5 = 0.4$$

$$\$39 \times 0.4 = \$15.60$$

$$\$39.00 - \$15.60 = \$23.40$$

Since I did the math, I can see that the second t-shirt is actually cheaper, even though the original price was higher.

Changing the fraction to a decimal leads us to another important concept: *rounding*. **Rounding** is a method of reducing the number of digits in a number so that it is less precise, but is more convenient to use. For example, to change a fraction to a decimal, you divide the numerator by the denominator. 2/5 = 0.4, four tenths. That is a pretty easy number to work with. However, dividing 1/3 gives us a quotient of 0.3333333333... and on forever. The 3s just keep repeating infinitely. To come up with a usable number, rounding rules need to be applied. To round a number to one decimal place (like 0.4), you look at the number immediately to the right of the place-holder that you want to round to. If the number is between 0 and 4, you drop the remaining digits and leave the number in the tenths place as it is. This is called rounding down. If the digit is between 5 and 9, you add one to the digit in the tenths place. This is called rounding up. In this case, the number in the 100ths place is a 3. Three is between 0 and 4, so you leave the 3 in the tenths place alone. The rounding process results in a 0.3. Although rounding leaves you with a number that is not as precise as your original result (0.333333333), it allows you to perform calculations that would be difficult, if not impossible.

In many health care applications, converting to a decimal makes a fraction easier to use. Let us say the city of Midville, Florida has three hospitals—two are larger facilities, and one is smaller. Of all the admissions last year, very few patients had a principal diagnosis of MRSA, a kind of bacterial infection that is difficult to treat with antibiotics.

TAKE AWAY •·········

Convert fractions into decimals by dividing the numerator by the denominator.

Rounding Reducing the number of digits in a number to make it easier to use.

Facility	2015 Admissions	2015 MRSA Cases
Midville General Hospital	14,065	2
Midville Lutheran Hospital	4,023	1
University of Midville Medical Center	12,200	1

What fraction (part of the whole) of patients in all three Midville hospitals had MRSA?

We know how to set up the fraction for each: $\dfrac{2}{14,065} + \dfrac{1}{4,203} + \dfrac{1}{12,200}$. But we would not want to try to find the common denominator of all these fractions in order to add them together. It would be much easier (though *slightly* less precise) to convert each fraction to a decimal, then add the decimals. Let us look at the math:

Facility	Numerator (MRSA Cases)		Denominator (Total Patients)		Quotient	Rounding
Midville General Hospital	2	÷	14,065	=	0.00014219694	0.00014
Midville Lutheran Hospital	1	÷	4023	=	0.00024857072	0.00025
University of Midville Medical Center	1	÷	12,200	=	0.00008196721	0.00008
Total	4	÷	30,288	=	0.00047273487	0.00047

● MATH REVIEW

If we say 0.00047 patients of all the patients in Midville had MRSA, how many people is that?

The 4 is in the 10,000s place, so we might say 4.7 infections for every 10,000 people. Or, we might say 47 of every 100,000 patients were treated for this infection.

Calculating the part of the whole of the patients in Midville who were treated for MRSA using fractions would be difficult; but when we convert the fractions to decimals and use rounding, we can see that 0.00047 of all the patients (30,288) in Midville had MRSA.

EXERCISE 2-2

Decimals

1. Convert the following fractions to decimals:

   a. $\dfrac{3}{8}$

   b. $13\dfrac{1}{2}$

   c. $7\dfrac{5}{16}$

   d. $\dfrac{1}{160}$

   e. $\dfrac{60}{10000}$

2. In the decimal 0.012358467, the digit 1 is in the _____ place.

3. In the decimal 0.193847, the digit 7 is in the _____ place.

4. Round each decimal to the tenths place. Then round each to the hundredths place. Then round to the thousandth place.

   a. 0.09513999
   b. 0.551031
   c. 1.342809

Percentages

Like a decimal, a percentage is also based on the number 10, or more precisely, the number 100. A **percentage** is the number of times something occurs out every 100 times. Percentages are useful because often, just stating the amount of something is confusing to the user. Presentation of the percentage standardizes the data so that unlike groups can be compared. One familiar example is the quiz grades you received for a class. If you answered 24 of 27 questions correctly on one quiz, and 30 of 35 questions right on another, which quiz did you score better on?

○ **Percentage** The number of times a thing occurs out of 100.

To calculate a percentage, divide the observations in the category by the total observations, and multiply by 100.

$$\frac{observations}{total\,observations} \times 100 = percentage$$

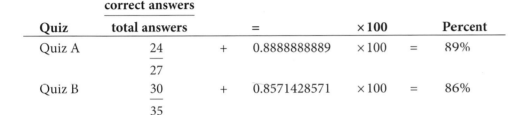

Quiz	correct answers / total answers		=	× 100		Percent
Quiz A	24/27	+	0.8888888889	× 100	=	89%
Quiz B	30/35	+	0.8571428571	× 100	=	86%

Since we standardized the data by looking at each score out of 100, we can see that the score on the first quiz was slightly better.

Now let us look at a simple health care application. Consider the question: *How many male and female patients were discharged in February this year compared to last year?* We can look at the difference (the variance) between the number of women and men in each period, as illustrated in Table 2-1, but the result may not be helpful.

TABLE 2-1			
VARIANCE BETWEEN NUMBER OF WOMEN AND MEN DISCHARGED IN FEBRUARY			
	FEBRUARY 2015	**FEBRUARY 2014**	**VARIANCE**
Males discharged	413	386	27
Females discharged	385	349	36
TOTAL	798	735	63

Just by looking at the table, we can see that more men than women were discharged in February both this year and last year. We can also see that discharges for both women and men have increased. It *appears* that there has been a larger increase in discharges of women (36) than in men (27). But is that true? To give a more accurate analysis of the activity in Table 2-1, we should also provide the percentage of observations and the percent variance.

For example, if we want to know what percent of the patients discharged in February 2014 were women, we would do the following:

$$\frac{349\ women\ discharged}{735\ total\ discharges} = 0.48246 \times 100 = 48\,\%$$

The calculation shows that 48% of the discharges in February 2014 were women. But what about the variance? How many *more* women were discharged in 2015? We can use the same calculation (observations divided by total observations) to determine the percent variance, showing exactly what happened:

$$\frac{\text{variance of women discharged}}{\text{total women discharged}} = \frac{36}{349} = 0.1032 \times 100 = 10\,\%$$

Table 2-2 expands the data to include the percentages. Now, it is clear that the total number of discharges has increased by 8.6%, the percentage of women increased by 10.3%, and the percentage of men increased by 7.0%. These are descriptive statistics, so we cannot say *why* there is a greater percentage increase in women patients than in men. We will have to examine this data over a longer period of time and look further into the types of illnesses and treatments that the patients have to understand the reason for the change, if it continues.

TAKE AWAY

Calculating percentages can allow you to estimate the impact of a decrease (or increase) in patient volume, which can tell you the number of personnel needed for a particular medical service.

TABLE 2-2

PERCENTAGE CHANGE IN NUMBER OF WOMEN AND MEN DISCHARGED IN FEBRUARY

PATIENTS DISCHARGED	FEBRUARY 2015		FEBRUARY 2014			
	NUMBER	% OF TOTAL	NUMBER	% OF TOTAL	VARIANCE	% VARIANCE
Male	413	52%	386	53%	27	7.0%
Female	385	48%	349	47%	36	10.3%
TOTAL	798	100%	735	100%	63	8.6%

Fractions, decimals, and percentages are closely related concepts, and in practice, you will need to be able to convert between these formats frequently. Box 2-1 summarizes the relationships between these concepts.

BOX 2-1   RELATIONSHIPS BETWEEN FRACTIONS, DECIMALS, AND PERCENTAGES

Fraction	Decimal	Percentage
1/100	0.01	1%
5/100, 1/20	0.05	5%
10/100, 1/10	0.1	10%
1/8	0.125	12.5%
25/100,5/25, 1/5	0.25	25%
50/100, 1/2	0.50	50%
100/100, 1	1.0	100%
125/100	1.25	125%
200/100	2.0	200%

TO CONVERT FROM A FRACTION TO A DECIMAL
Divide the numerator (top number) by the denominator (bottom number).

TO CONVERT FROM A DECIMAL TO A FRACTION
Divide the decimal number by the power of 10 that it represents, then simplify the fraction.

| BOX 2-1 | RELATIONSHIPS BETWEEN FRACTIONS, DECIMALS, AND PERCENTAGES—cont'd |

TO CONVERT FROM A DECIMAL TO A PERCENT
Multiply the decimal by 100, and add a percentage sign.

TO CONVERT FROM A PERCENT TO A DECIMAL
Divide the percentage by 100, and drop the percentage sign.

Stat Tip

Dividing the percentage by 100 results in moving the decimal point two places to the left. Once you are comfortable with this method, you may want to use it as a shortcut for conversions.

TO CONVERT FROM A FRACTION TO A PERCENTAGE
Divide the numerator by the denominator, then multiply the result by 100, and add a percentage sign.

TO CONVERT FROM A PERCENTAGE TO A FRACTION
Drop the percentage sign, then divide the decimal number by the power of 10 that it represents.

EXERCISE 2-3
Percentages

1. Calculate the following percentages:

   a. 10/50
   b. 49/100
   c. 17/1000
   d. 14/16
   e. 1810/2000

2. Convert the following percentages to decimals:

   a. 1%
   b. 10%
   c. 47%
   d. 0.5%

3. Convert the following to the simplest fraction:

   a. .5
   b. 0.98
   c. 0.333333333
   d. 1.75
   e. 90%
   f. 25%

RATIO, RATE, AND PROPORTION

Ratio

While fractions and decimals help to describe parts of numbers that are generally smaller than one, a ratio is more useful in comparing one group of numbers to another. Some of the vocabulary and concepts that you have learned about them can be recycled here to explain this statistical term.

A **ratio** is a comparison of two or more numbers using the same unit of measurement (time/dollars/weight). Ratios can be expressed with either a colon or a slash between the two numbers. As always, an example helps make this concept more understandable. One common ratio we use in the classroom is the ratio of students to teachers. Let us say in an average class, there are 23 students for every teacher. The ratio of students to teachers, then, is 23 to 1, or 23:1.

Another example is the number of nurses to patients on a unit. If a particular floor is very busy and the nurses are short-staffed, we might see a ratio of 1:6, or one nurse to every six patients. In the ICU where nursing care is critical, the facility would aim for a ratio of 1:2 or even 1:1 nurse per patient.

Hospital A treated a total of 47 patients at its Saturday morning clinic. Thirty-two of the patients were female, while 15 were male. The ratio of females to males was 32:15 or 32/15. This is useful in giving an overall impression of the magnitude of the similarity or differences between the groups compared; in this case, we can see that there were more women treated this Saturday—a lot more! Using your knowledge of rounding and reducing fractions, a 30:15 ratio would be expressed as 2:1 in its simplest form.

When working with a ratio, pay close attention to the order. 32:15 is not the same as 15:32! Also, if the units are of different magnitudes (example: minutes vs. hours for time), you need to convert them to be the same unit to make a comparison. Let us say we are looking at two people, Althea and Zinnia, who are both coding medical records. If Althea codes 6 records every 30 minutes (6:30), then reducing the ratio we could say she codes 1 record every 5 minutes, or 1:5. Zinnia, on the other hand, codes 13 records an hour, or 13:1. Who is faster? We would have to convert Zinnia's magnitude to minutes—or Althea's to hours—to find out.

Rate

Rates are comparisons of two numbers that are measured with *different* units of measurement, calculated as a numerator divided by a denominator. To make an example that is close to your study, you might want to calculate how many minutes it takes you to work through examples in the book. If you can do three examples every 10 minutes (or three examples/10 minutes), you can use the calculation to realize it takes you about $3\frac{1}{3}$ minutes per example. If you know that you have 12 examples to work through, you can use the rate to find out how many minutes the exercises will take.

Rates need to be labeled with the unit that is being measured. In this example, the unit would be "minutes per example." If we were comparing the dollars in DRG (diagnosis-related group) reimbursement for each DRG, the unit would be "dollars per case." If we looked at the number of malpractice claims in the hospital by month, it would be claims/month. Note that this is different than ratios that are expressed as simply one number compared to another, because in ratios, the units of measure are the same.

Rates are very, very common in health statistics and data analytics. Because there is often an element of time involved, facilities frequently use rates to determine how they are performing. For any given month or year, they might examine birth rates, death rates, rates of infection, rates the physicians consulted with one another—just to name a few. We will look at the kind of rates used for benchmarking more closely in Chapter 5.

○ Ratio A comparison of two or more numbers using the same unit of measurement.

● ICU Intensive care unit.

● MATH REVIEW

There are 60 minutes in 1 hour. Althea's ratio is 6 records to 30 minutes (6:30), so we can multiply that by 2, finding she codes 12 records every 60 minutes. Zinnia's coding ratio is 13 records to 60 minutes (13:60), so she is slightly faster.

○ Rate A value in relation to a different unit.

● DRG Diagnosis-related group.

● MATH REVIEW

If you can do one example every $3\frac{1}{3}$ minutes, how long does it take to do 12? 12 examples $\times 3\frac{1}{3}$ min $= 40$ minutes.

Proportion

Proportions are expressed as two equal ratios. ½ cup = 2/4 cups. Proportions are useful in figuring out unknown values when you know one ratio and want to determine what one of the other two variables would be.

Let us say that it is a hospital policy to make sure there are always three nurses for every patient on the med-surg floor. This hospital has found that if the nurses become more outnumbered than that (e.g., 4:1), the quality of care suffers, and if there are fewer than that (e.g., 2:1), the nurses have quite a bit of downtime. So, if today we have 24 patients and we want to make sure we have the right amount of nurses, how do we set up the proportion? In this case, some basic algebra helps us solve the problem.

○ **Proportion** The relation of four quantities in two equal ratios, where the first quantity divided by the second equals the third divided by the fourth.

$$\frac{1\,\text{nurse}}{3\,\text{patients}} = \frac{x\,\text{nurses}}{24\,\text{patients}}$$

To solve the problem, you can use a trick called cross-multiplication:

$$\frac{1\ \text{nurse}}{3\ \text{patients}} \diagdown\!\!\!\!\diagup \frac{x\ \text{nurses}}{24\ \text{patients}}$$

$$3x = 24$$

$$x = 8$$

To meet quality standards, we would have to staff this floor with 8 nurses.

Proportions can be either direct or inverse. A direct proportion is one in which there is an increase in one quantity when there is an increase in the other—or a decrease in one quantity when there is a decrease in another. We might observe that as the number of nurses per floor increases, so does the number of positive comments per satisfaction survey. This is a direct proportion. An inverse proportion is the opposite: when there is an increase in one quantity, there is a decrease in the other. As the number of flu shots per month increases, for instance, the number of cases of flu per month decreases.

Table 2-3 compares rate, ratio, and proportion.

TABLE 2-3			
COMPARISON OF RATIO, RATE, AND PROPORTION			
STATISTIC	**UNITS OF MEASUREMENT**	**APPEARANCE**	**EXAMPLE**
Rate	Different	Expressed as a quotient or with a colon between the two variables	A family physician sees 3 patients every hour. 3:1 hour or $\dfrac{3\ \text{patients}}{1\ \text{hour}}$
Ratio	Same	Expressed as a quotient or with a colon between the two variables	7 of every 10 patients the physician sees are over the age of 60. 7:10 patients or $\dfrac{7\ \text{patients over age 60}}{10\ \text{patients}}$
Proportion	Different	Expressed as two ratios	A medical practice has 4 PAs and 9 doctors. The proportion is $\dfrac{4\,\text{PAs}}{13\,\text{clinicians}} = \dfrac{9\,\text{doctors}}{13\,\text{clinicians}}$

EXERCISE 2-4
Ratio, Rate, and Proportion

1. Alana can code 8 charts in 1 hour. What is the ratio of minutes to charts?

2. The group practice's policy is that for every 3 physicians in the group, there should be one medical assistant (MA). If there are 12 physicians in the group, how many MAs should the practice employ?

3. A radiology center on the east side of town performs 12 X-rays a day. A larger, competing center on the west side of town performs 30 X-rays a day. What is the simplest ratio of east side X-rays performed to west side X-rays?

VOLUME, FREQUENCY, AND FREQUENCY DISTRIBUTION

In the last chapter, we talked about how descriptive statistics are used to give an overall impression of a group of data. As an HIM professional, you may be required to (numerically) describe patients, employees, diseases, procedures, or any number of health care events. The descriptions may include ages, salaries, outcomes, and many other values. Very simply, those descriptions will be answers to a series of questions:

How many are there?
What are the characteristics of the group?
How similar/different are the subgroups of characteristics?
What are the relationships between the subgroups?

The individual descriptions for each question (100 patients; 10 are 4 years old; 6 are 37 years old; we pay graduate nurses $45,000/year; 4 patients deceased last month) are the values that can answer the real question: *What is the variable for this particular observation?* The first sets of descriptive statistics that we cover will help answer those questions.

The very first, and simplest, numeric description of a group of data is its volume, or total, and it is one of the most common questions asked by managers and administrators. They want to know: *how many?*

- The hospital admitted 7593 patients last year.
- There were 162 tonsillectomies performed over the last 5 years.
- A physician practice currently employs 26 professionals.

Notice that these are totals for each example. To determine the total number of patients treated, for example, an administrator would ask *how many* admissions or discharges occurred during a certain period.

Volume

Volume The count of an activity or value.

Some questions that ask *how many* are asking about **volume**, the count of an activity or value. Volume is an important measure for defining activity and for comparing activity from one period to the next or among departments or facilities. It can tell us a lot about how much of an activity we are doing, or how much more (or less) we are doing compared to other times or other facilities.

Say, for example, you and the kid next door decide to operate a lemonade stand. At the end of the month, you count the money the stand collected, totaling $500. This is the volume for July, describing the total activity for the month. After toasting to your success with an ice-cold, fresh-squeezed lemonade, you find out that the stand two blocks away made $700 in July. Calculating volume tells us how much activity we did, and comparing volumes tells us how much activity we might have done.

In health care, we can provide volume figures on any type of data by counting the total number of observations of the particular data element, or by counting the number of observations in a particular category. So, we can count the revenues collected, the number of female patients, the number of Asian patients, the number of patients who were age 65, the number of tonsillectomies, and the number of patients discharged on a particular date.

Say the manager asks, "*What was the volume of discharges last month?*" She wants to know the total number of discharges (how many) occurred. But to answer a volume question, we need to know more about what specific volume is being requested. In particular, we need to know the following:

1. The month: the first and last dates, including the year
2. The specific type of patient (inpatient or outpatient)
3. If there are any services that must be included or excluded (e.g., emergency department or same day surgery; newborns or adults)

Say that the manager answers those questions like this: *I want to know the volume of discharges in September of 2015 for all adult inpatients.* Now we know that we need to count the number of discharges of adult inpatients that occurred from 9/1/2015 through 9/30/2015. The next question is what constitutes an adult? Let us say that our hospital considers all patients over the age of 16 as adults. There are two steps to this analysis. We need to count only September, 2015, and we need to omit any patients under the age of 16. So, we can sort the database by discharge date, then sort the month of September by patient age. Then, count the number of patients who are age 17 and older.

In an electronic record environment, the software has usually been programmed to report the most common volumes needed for management and administrative purposes. Some common volumes include number of discharges by date, diagnosis, procedure, attending physician, and surgeon. Often, variations on those volumes can be queried if there is no standard report available.

Stat Tip ·································

Counting can be done manually. It can also be done by using a formula in an electronic spreadsheet. In Excel, the counting formula is =COUNT(RANGE) for numerical values, such as counting the number of admission type codes on a list, and =COUNTA(RANGE) for alphanumeric values, such as counting the number of names on a list.

Frequency

Where volume tells us the amount of an activity, **frequency** describes the number of times a specific value for a variable occurs. If you wanted to know how many people in the class are male, for example, you would be asking about the frequency of men in the group. Looking at the class roster in Figure 2-3 as a sample, the variable is gender, the value is male, and the frequency is 6 times in this class of 23.

Statisticians sometimes talk about an *absolute frequency*, the total number of values for the variable being measured. In the class roster example, the absolute frequency is all 23 students. **Relative frequency** is calculated as a percentage and is described with percentages. The relative frequency is the observed frequency of a value divided by the absolute frequency. In other words, it is the ratio of the number of values in a particular category to the total number of values in that group. It can be described also as a

Frequency The total number of occurrences of a value.

Relative frequency The observed frequency of a value divided by the absolute frequency (the total).

Class Roster		
Name	Age	Gender
Alex	19	Male
Amanda	21	Female
Ashley	19	Female
Brittany	20	Female
Elizabeth	19	Female
Emily	21	Female
Hannah	23	Female
Jack	20	Male
Jessica	20	Female
John	33	Male
Kayla	19	Female
Lauren	20	Female
Margaret	27	Female
Marion	19	Female
Megan	21	Female
Rick	26	Male
Rob	19	Male
Samantha	22	Female
Sarah	20	Female
Scott	25	Male
Stephanie	22	Female
Sue	29	Female
Taylor	22	Female

Figure 2-3 Class roster.

proportion, a part of a whole, or as a coin toss. Let us look again at our class roster. How can you tell the relative frequency of *males* in the class? It is the observed frequency, which is 6, divided by the absolute frequency, 23, or 26%.

Frequency Distribution

Sometimes answering the question *how many* does not give the user enough meaningful information. For example, the instructor of this course might think that most of her students have earned a passing grade. She could just count how many students got a 70, how many got a 71, how many got an 80, etc. That would give us the volume of students who received a particular score. However, that just gives us a long list of data that is not meaningful.

Remember that grades and salaries and ages are examples of continuous, ratio data. Although they most commonly appear as a whole number (e.g., 90, $45,000, 7 years old), they are, nevertheless, continuous. A common way to analyze age and other continuous data is with a **frequency distribution**. Frequency distributions can include either grouped or ungrouped data. A grouped frequency distribution takes the categories of the variable and groups those categories into equal ranges. Each of these smaller groupings of data is called a **class**.

Each class must be mutually exclusive, meaning that any value that is assigned to a class can fit in one and only one class. The *class limits* (upper and lower) are the

○ **Frequency distribution** The organization of data into tabular format using mutually exclusive classes and frequencies.

○ **Class** A group of values in a frequency distribution.

TABLE 2-4

CLASS GRADES IN A FREQUENCY DISTRIBUTION

CLASS	LOWER LIMIT	UPPER LIMIT	CLASS INTERVAL	CLASS WIDTH (OR SIZE)	VALUES	FREQUENCY
A	90	100	90–100	11	90, 90, 93, 97, 100	5
B	80	89	80–89	10	81, 83, 85, 85, 86, 88, 88, 89	8
C	70	79	70–79	10	70, 71, 73, 75, 75, 78, 78, 79	8
D	60	69	60–69	10	62	1
F	0	59	0–59	60	49	1

values that separate one class from another. For example, course grades are tradition-ally divided into groups or classes of A, B, C, D, and F. The class limits for each are A (90–100), B (80–89), C (70–79), D (60–69) and F (<60). The upper and lower limits together are called a *class interval*. Look at Table 2-4. Notice that there are no overlaps in any of the classes—they are mutually exclusive. An 80 goes in the B class and cannot be categorized as an A or a C. If the groups were A (90–100), B (80–90), C (70–80), D (60–70), and F (0–60), you have groupings that overlap, and an 80 could be either a B or a C. Obviously, that system just will not be acceptable for grades and certainly not for categorizing any type of data.

With each student's grade grouped into this frequency distribution, the instructor can see that yes, most students did earn a passing grade. Out of the 23 students in the class, eight received a C, another eight got a B, and five got As. Since $8 + 8 + 5 = 21$, 21 of the 23 students passed.

Let us look at an example in health care. How can a frequency distribution answer the *how many* question better than volume? The nursing managers may be telling adminis-tration that there are a lot of patients who require interpreters. Or that lately they have too many geriatric patients, putting pressure on the nursing staff to expand the number of nurses with geriatric competency and challenging the facility's resources. Now, we could just count how many patients there were of each age—how many 1 year olds, how many 2 year olds, etc. But again, that would leave us with a long, unhelpful list of data; grouping the patients into age ranges would make it much easier to see how much of the hospital's resources are being utilized to treat certain patients. If the ages of our patients range from 1 to 100, we can group those ages into five ranges of 20 ages each, 10 ranges of 10 ages each, or 20 ranges of five ages each, as follows:

5 Ranges of 20 Ages	10 Ranges of 10 Ages	20 Ranges of 5 Ages	
0–20	0–10	0–5	51–55
21–40	11–20	6–10	56–60
41–60	21–30	11–15	61–65
61–80	31–40	16–20	66–70
81–100	41–50	21–25	71–75
	51–60	26–30	76–80
	61–70	31–35	81–85
	71–80	36–40	86–90
	81–90	41–45	91–95
	91–100	46–50	96–100

Which grouping is best? It depends on what we are trying to determine. Let us think about why we are doing this analysis. At the moment, we just want to get a sense of the ages of our patients, to answer the question *where is our concentration of patients*? For that purpose, we can use the five ranges of 20 ages grouping. In the table below, the volume column is the count of patients in each age range, and the cumulative frequency is a running total of all classes.

Age	Volume	Cumulative Frequency	Relative Frequency
0-20	78	**78**	$78/1095 \times 100 = 7.1\%$
21-40	173	$(78 + 173) = \mathbf{251}$	$251/1095 \times 100 = 22.9\%$
41-60	251	$(78 + 173 + 251) = \mathbf{502}$	$502/1095 \times 100 = 45.8\%$
61-80	265	$(78 + 173 + 251 + 502) = \mathbf{767}$	$767/1095 \times 100 = 70.0\%$
81-100	328	$(78 + 173 + 251 + 502 + 767) = \mathbf{1095}$	$1095/1095 \times 100 = 100\%$

What does this distribution tell us? We see very few patients under the age of 20. Over half of our patients are over the age of 60. So, in terms of hospital services, it seems as though we have been concentrating on the elderly population. Further analysis is necessary to determine whether increasing services would be helpful. We would need to look at the competition in the marketplace and the demographic profile of the *catchment area* (the geographic area that the hospital serves).

EXERCISE 2-5

1. The children's wing has 25 male patients and 16 female patients. What is the absolute frequency? What is the relative frequency of males? Of females? What is the ratio of boys to girls in its simplest form?

2. While looking at salaries of nurses at the hospital, you find a range from a low of $25,000 to a high of $80,000. How many classes would you have if you broke them into class widths of $5000?

MEASURES OF CENTRAL TENDENCY

Measures of central tendency can be remembered as the 3 M's: mean, median and mode. You probably recognize the term mean as being synonymous with the word average. Your average for the course determines your grade; you may decide to browse careers on their average salary; and everyone wants to be above average. But do you know what an average is and how to calculate one? Each of the measures of central tendency aims to find a single value that best represents the rest of the data. Do you know when it makes sense to use the mean to describe your data and when you should use one of those other M's?

Mean

Mean The sum of the values divided by the total number of observations.

The **mean** is the sum of the values in the data that you are measuring divided by the total number of observations. Synonyms for the mean are the average, the arithmetic mean, and the expected value. This calculation helps to answer the question: *what is the usual number or amount?* For example, you have one course that has 5 exams. You earn a 90, a 0, a 90, an 80, and a 100. The average for the course is $90 + 0 + 90 + 80 + 100 \div 5$, and $360 \div 5 = 72$.

In any group of data, there is only one mean, and that calculation can be affected by extreme values, called **outliers**. The exam on which you scored a zero (the outlier) has a huge impact on your average. Students sometimes are unaware of the effect of an outlier. If you had gotten another 80 instead of a zero, your average would have been $90 + 80 + 90 + 80 + 100 \div 5$, and $440 \div 5 = 88$.

> **Outlier** An extreme value in a set of data.

> **TAKE AWAY** •·········
>
> To calculate the mean, add the sum of the group of numbers, and divide the sum by the number of items in the group.

Stat Tip ···

Calculate the mean easily in Excel using the average formula: = average(cell range).

> **ALOS** Average length of stay.

Outliers certainly influence important statistics like average length of stay (ALOS) where most patients stay 2–3 days, but a few stay up to 90 days, greatly skewing the mean. Facilities regularly use ALOS to determine the amount of resources their patients require. We will examine ALOS in greater detail in Chapter 4 on administrative data, but here is a simple example. The table below lists the lengths of stay for women who delivered babies by Caesarean section.

Patient	Length of Stay (LOS)
Kraut, Helene	2
Smith, Belinda	3
Serafin, Natalia	2
Jones, Janice	4
Rothschild, Pauline	32
Total days	**43**
ALOS	**8.6**

Just taking the mean LOS of these five patients, we calculate an ALOS of 8.6 days per patient. But is 8.6 really representative of the average patient's stay after a C-section? Certainly not; none of the other patients in this data set even stayed more than 4 days. Here is another example: Dr. Garcia performs a variety of general surgeries, but his highest volume is the cholecystectomy, the surgical removal of the gallbladder. Here is a set of observations regarding Dr. Garcia's volume:

> **LOS** Length of stay.

January	12 cases
February	12 cases
March	12 cases
April	13 cases
May	12 cases
June	2 cases
Total	63 cases

Now consider the question: *what is the average number of cases per month by Dr. Garcia in the first half of 2016?* If we use the arithmetic mean, the answer is 10.5 (63 cases divided by 6 months). Does that make sense? Of course not. Dr. Garcia usually performs between 12 and 13 procedures. He has not performed less than 12 procedures, until June. Fortunately, we can use one of our other M's to get a better idea of how long these patients *usually* stay.

Median

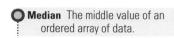

Median The middle value of an ordered array of data.

The second measure of central tendency is called the *median*. The **median** is the number that represents the middle of an ordered array of the data you are examining. Another way to state the definition is to say that 50% of the values are above the median, and 50% of the values are below it. A median is useful because, unlike the mean, it is not affected by extreme values. However, like the mean, there is only one. To determine the median value, you must place the values in numerical order from lowest to highest (or highest to lowest).

You might have noticed that the median instead of mean salaries are often reported because of the influence of very low or very high examples. For example, the Quick Facts about health careers on the Bureau of Labor Statistics Occupational Outlook Handbook site (http://www.bls.gov/ooh/Management/Medical-and-health-services-managers.htm) includes the median pay for each career.

Let us take the previous grades (90, 0, 90, 80, and 100). When we put them in order, you can easily see that the middle grade is a 90. At this point, you can see that the median (90) would be the same regardless of whether the lowest grade was an 80 or a zero. (Although interesting to note, it is probably not a negotiating tool to get a better grade!)

What if you had an even set of numbers? Half of your samples will be divisible by two, so consequently, the middle number will not be in the sample. An example of this would be six grades instead of five. Look at 100, 90, 90, 80, 80, and 80. The two middle grades are 90 and 80. In order to calculate the median, add the two middle grades together and divide by two. So, $90° + °80/2° = °85$. In this case, the median is 85.

Let us go back again to Dr. Garcia's surgeries. To determine the median for our example data set, arrange the data in numerical order from lowest to highest:

June	2 cases
February	12 cases
January	12 cases
March	12 cases
May	12 cases
April	13 cases
Total	63 cases

There are 63 observations. The median is the midpoint in the list of observations: in this case, observation #32. Counting down from the top of the list, the value associated with observation #32 is 12. Therefore, the median number of cases for Dr. Garcia in the first 6 months of 2013 is 12. Note that there are an odd number of observations. If there were an even number of observations, we would take the average of the two middle observations. So, assuming there were 64 observations, we would average the value of observations 32 and 33. When we calculate the arithmetic mean and the results do not make sense based on what we know the data otherwise reflects, we can use the median to give us more insight into the distribution of the data. For further clarification we can use our third M, the mode.

Mode

The last of the measures of central tendency is the **mode**. The mode is the most frequently occurring observation in your sample. Using the 6 grades in the median example (100, 90, 90, 80, 80 and 80), you can see that you have one 100, two 90s, and three 80s. Because the 80 grades occur three times (more than two 90s or one 100), 80 is the mode for these grades. Because the mode is simply the most frequently occurring, no calculation is needed. However, unlike the mean or median, there can be more than one mode. An instructor might look at the class grades and see that he has 5 As, 8 Bs, 8 Cs, 1 D, and 1 F. In this case, the modes would be B and C because they both have the same highest number of grades. This would be an example of a bimodal (bi- = two) distribution of grades. If there were three highest values, it would be called trimodal (tri- = three). It is also possible that no mode exists. So the mode is different from the mean and median in that they will always have one and only one value, while the mode can have none, one, or more than one value. In a large group of observations, a mode with many observations may indicate a strong preference or tendency of the group. Because the mode is not a numerical calculation, it is possible that the group will have no mode (because all of the observations are at a single value). The lack of a mode is not inherently important.

> **Mode** The most frequently occurring observation in a set of data.

The mode answers questions like *what is the most common number of procedures performed by Dr. Garcia each month*? In our example above, the most common number of procedures performed is 12—the same number as the median. In this case, the median and the mode are the same—casting further suspicion on the usefulness of the arithmetic mean in this group of data. In this example, the median and the mode are better descriptions of Dr. Garcia's volume than the arithmetic mean.

However, the arithmetic mean does alert us to an anomaly in Dr. Garcia's volume. In reviewing the data, we can see the sharp drop in volume that occurred in July. Administrators may be concerned that Dr. Garcia has decided to perform his surgeries at another hospital. A simple phone call to the medical staff office or the health information management department may reveal that Dr. Garcia is on vacation for a month and will resume surgeries in August. A confirmation call to the scheduling department may yield the information that Dr. Garcia is already fully booked for the first two weeks in August.

Although this example is certainly simple, changes from month to month in statistical indicators such as the case-mix index (CMI) or average volume should trigger investigations into the reason for the change. Thus, statistics can be extremely helpful in monitoring activities and highlighting changes before they become problematic.

Table 2-5 compares the three M's of central tendency.

TABLE 2-5				
THE THREE M'S OF CENTRAL TENDENCY				
CENTRAL TENDENCY	**SYNONYMS?**	**HOW MANY POSSIBLE?**	**AFFECTED BY EXTREME VALUES?**	**IS ORDER NECESSARY TO CALCULATE?**
Mean	Average	One	Yes	No
Median	None	One	No	Yes
Mode	None	None, one, more than one	No	Yes

BRIEF CASE

FINDING MEAN, MEDIAN, AND MODE

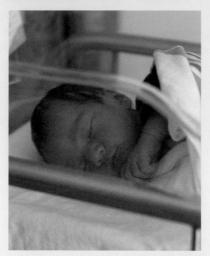

Sasha is trying to determine the hospital equipment and staffing needs for maternity care. Since newborn stays are largely determined by the LOS of the mother, newborn statistics are often reviewed in conjunction with obstetrical delivery data. The table below shows the LOS for newborns discharged over the course of a week. What are the mean, median, and mode for this data set?

LOS: NEWBORNS, DISCHARGED 4/15–4/22

LOS	Number of Discharges	Total Days
1 day	3	3
2 days	7	14
3 days	7	21
4 days	2	8
5 days	1	5
6 days	0	0
7 days	1	7
	21	58

Adjusted Mean

Another way to look at the central tendency of data in which the mean, median, and mode do not agree is to adjust the mean.

To adjust the mean of a set of data, we remove some of the data: the outliers. Typically, we remove not only the outliers on one end but also the corresponding number (or percentage) of observations on the other end: highest and lowest or largest and smallest. For example, removing the first two and last two observations in Dr. Garcia's surgery list gives us 59 observations over 5 months (note that June is now eliminated). Thus, the adjusted mean is 11.8: much closer to the 12 per month that we were expecting.

The purpose of adjusting the mean is only to get a sense of how unusual the outliers really are. Up to 5% of the highest and 5% of the lowest is generally acceptable. In the absence of policies or conventions, it is up to the presenter (the analyzer of the data) to determine what percentage should be adjusted. However, a clear explanation of the adjustment must accompany the report. The take away for all of the coverage of central tendency is that these measures are seeking a way to describe the similarities in your group of data. Each of the measures offers a different number (or different numbers) to give you a snapshot of a characteristic that gives a quick idea of what your group looks like.

Stat Tip ···

It may be useful to provide the report both with and without the adjustment so that the user can see exactly what impact the adjustment had on the reported data.

EXERCISE 2-6
Measures of Central Tendency

1. A home health nurse visited three patients on Monday, four on Tuesday, two on Wednesday, and four on Thursday. What is the average number of patients he saw on those four days? Provide your answer to the hundredths decimal place.

2. Over 12 months, an acute care facility compiled a report of the number of patients transferred by month to a neighboring skilled nursing facility (SNF): 3, 10, 10, 11, 6, 10, 12, 11, 15, 8, 9, and 6.

   a. What is the mean number of patients transferred per month?
   b. What is the median?
   c. What is the mode?
   d. Which outliers would you remove to calculate the adjusted mean? What is your calculation?

DISPERSION

The last basic math concept that needs to be addressed is that of **dispersion**, or the spread of the data. Are all of your values close together or are they spread apart from each other? Dispersion deals with differences, not similarities. For example, a student with grades that are 82, 81, 79, 85, and 83 has grades that are fairly close together. Another student has grades of 82, 67, 98, 76, and 32—quite a bit of difference among those grades!

> ⬤ **Dispersion** The spread of the data.

One of the simplest measures to describe dispersion is called the **range**. The range is the difference between the lowest and highest (or highest and lowest) observation. The statistical range for the first student is 85–79 (or 79–85) with a range of six points. The second student's grades range from a high of 98 to a low of 32. That student's range is 98–32 = 66. The range is a simple, but crude method of looking at how different the scores are. You can see it in three formats: highest to lowest, lowest to highest, or the difference between the two.

> ⬤ **Range** The difference between the lowest and highest (or highest and lowest) observation.

Interquartile Range

If a simple range is used, extreme values can sway a truer measure of spread. Interquartile and semi-interquartile ranges are used in health care when extreme values (outliers) are present and the data analyst wants a less influenced picture of the data.

Fractiles are a means of dividing the data into fractional percentages. A *decile* is a type of fractile dividing the data into percentages of 10, while *quartiles* divide the data into percentages of 25 (quarters). Most commonly, a measure of spread that is used with the median is the semi-interquartile range. The interquartile range and semi-interquartile range are two measures that use the median, take out the influence of extreme values, and help provide a cleaner picture of your data.

Using the data below, we can divide our 20 observations of patient lengths of stay into quartiles. Each will have values that have 25% of the values. We can then observe that any factor of 25 (i.e., 25, 50, 75) is above or below a particular value (Figure 2-4).

Patient	LOS
A. Booker	8
B. McCall	3
C. Rossman	46
D. Elias	6
E. Roman	1
F. Shumacher	3
G. Ashton	17
H. Dorrance	19
I. Edwards	3
J. Frank	4
K. Goode	1
L. Moore	2
M. Nunez	10
N. Orville	5
O. Pau	7
P. Quigley	3
R. Tamaka	12
S. Underwood	4
T. Weiner	1
U. Yellen	2

The interquartile range is a measure of variation that is the absolute value of the difference between the first and third quartiles. In this example, the interquartile range is 9–3, or 6 days. If the interquartile range is divided in half, it gives a statistic that gives an approximation of how far the scores spread from the median. For the example used, this would be 6/2 = +/− 3.

Variance

While central tendency looks at what the values have in common, another type of statistic, the variance, looks at their differences. Variance is a measure of how different the values are from each other. A simple measure of variance is used in budgeting when managers compare their projected allotments to what was actually spent. In this use, variances may be favorable or unfavorable. An over-spending is obviously unfavorable, while staying under budget is favorable. This concept could also extend to increases/decreases in expected or target values for admissions or deaths. An increase in admissions from one period to another is likely favorable, while an increase in the number of deaths is probably unfavorable. (Thus, favorability is somewhat subjective.)

But variance is also a term that is used to describe another important statistical concept: the difference between the calculated mean of a group of data and each individual observation. What the variance helps us understand here is *how different is each item/ patient from the average for the group as a whole?* To calculate this variance, we take the average of the squared differences from the mean.

Let us look at a couple of examples to get a feel for this type of variance:

Emily's grades are fairly close together: 82, 81, 79, 85, and 83.

Amanda's grades have a wider dispersion: 82, 67, 98, 76, and 32.

Step 1: Order the observed values from lowest to highest

	Patient	Length of stay
1	E. Roman	1
2	T. Weiner	1
3	L. Moore	2
4	U. Yellen	2
5	B. McCall	3
6	F. Shumacher	3
7	I. Edwards	3
8	P. Quigley	3
9	J. Frank	4
10	S. Underwood	4
11	N. Orville	5
12	K. Goode	6
13	D. Elias	6
14	O. Pau	7
15	A. Booker	8
16	M. Nunez	10
17	R. Tamaka	12
18	G. Ashton	17
19	H. Dorrance	19
20	C. Rossman	46

Step 2: Divide the ordered values into 4 groups

Step 3: Starting with the 50% value (the median), you can see that half of your values are above and below this number. In this array, the 10th and 11th values are 4 and 5, so the median is 4+5/2 = 4.5. The 25% quartile is determined by observing the 5th and 6th values 3 and 3, so the first quartile is 3 (25% of the values are 3 or less). The 75% quartile is 8 and 10, so the 75% quartile is 8+10/2 = 9. 75% of the values are less than 9.

Figure 2-4 Finding a fractile: quartiles.

Score	Score Minus Mean	Difference	Squared
79	79 − 82	−3	9
81	81 − 82	−1	1
82	82 − 82	0	0
83	83 − 82	1	1
85	85 − 82	3	9
		Sum	**20**

To calculate variance, we need to first obtain the mean. For Emily, we calculate 82 + 81 + 79 + 85 + 83 = 410 ÷ 5 = 82. Emily's grade average is 82. Next, we need to determine what the difference is between each score and the mean for all of the scores. Then, we square each sum and add them all together.

This sum is 20, so the last step is to divide the sum by 5, and 20/5 = 4. The variance for this particular student's scores is 4. We will give additional meaning to this number in a moment, but for now, the 4 represents the average difference between Emily's scores and the mean.

> ## Stat Tip ···
>
> You might ask why we squared the differences from the mean. Take a look at the sum of the differences above: it is zero! The only way to get an amount that we can work with is to square each result (do not worry, we will "unsquare" it later in our calculations).

Let us take a look at Amanda's grades with the huge range in her scores, and we will go ahead and calculate a variance.

$$32 + 67 + 76 + 82 + 98 = 355.355 \div 5 = 71 \text{ for her mean (average)}$$

Score	Score Minus Mean	Difference	Squared
32	32–71	−39	1521
67	67–71	−4	16
76	76–71	5	25
82	82–71	11	121
98	98–71	27	729
		Sum	**2412**

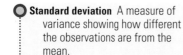

MATH REVIEW

Note that we rounded this number down.

Add the sum of the squares: $1521 + 16 + 25 + 121 + 729 = 2412$. Dividing 2412 by $5 = 482.4$. The variance for the first sample is 4, while the second is 482. This is a numerical measure of just how different these two students are in the consistency of performing the same on the tests that they have taken.

There are two important points:

1. If all of the scores are the same, the variance would be zero! And that would mean that the scores are not different from each other at all.
2. You should know that variance is seldom used by itself, but it is most often used as a means to calculate our final statistic, standard deviation. So let us move on to this often misunderstood but important statistic.

Standard Deviation

Although range and variance give rough ideas of the differences in the high and low values in your data, there is another statistic that gives another perspective and even more information about your sample. **Standard deviation** is the square root of the variance and is represented by the Greek letter sigma, σ. Standard deviation is a measure of how spread out our numbers are. It tells you if they are clumped together (a small standard deviation) or spread far apart (a large standard deviation).

To continue using our examples with student test scores, Emily's standard deviation would be the square root of 5, or 2.23, rounded off to ± 2 (note that square roots can be positive or negative). The second student's standard deviation would be the square root of 603, or 24.55, rounded off to ± 25. The higher the standard deviation, the more varied the data tends to be from the average.

The concept of standard deviation is based on a random sample, and it is used to predict the probability of future events with a specified degree of confidence. You may have heard of the bell curve (Figure 2-5), which is the classic representation of a normal distribution. A normal distribution uses standard deviation to show how scores are expected to cluster around the calculated average of a sample or population.

Standard deviation A measure of variance showing how different the observations are from the mean.

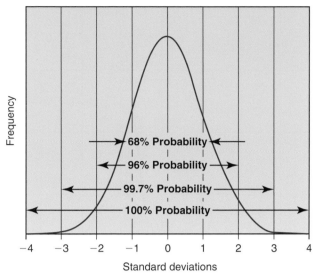

Figure 2-5 A bell curve.

Again, using our first example, there is a 68% probability that Emily's scores would be within ± 2 of her average (82 + 2 = 84, and 82 − 2 = 80). So the scores of 80 to 84 are within 1 standard deviation from the mean. Two standard deviations from the mean could be calculated by adding and subtracting 2 more from each of these results (78 − 86), which gives us a 96% probability of including all the scores.

Amanda has been much less consistent, and therefore, her results are much more difficult to predict. She had a standard deviation of ± 25. One standard deviation for Amanda would be ± 25 from the mean of 71. That would give 46–96, and 2 standard deviations would be 21–122! Notice in Figure 2-6 that the larger the standard deviation, the flatter the bell curve, while the smaller it is, the more peaked it appears.

Stat Tip ··

Perhaps you are not relishing the task of calculating standard deviation by hand. Fortunately, it can be accomplished fairly easily using Excel.

1. Click a cell directly below the column of numbers that you want a standard deviation for and type the formula = STDEV([*cell range*]).

2. Highlight that entire column of values that you wish to examine and press enter. Your calculated standard deviation will immediately appear. (You could also type each value in individually; each number must be separated from the next with a comma, and you will need to end with a close parenthesis.)

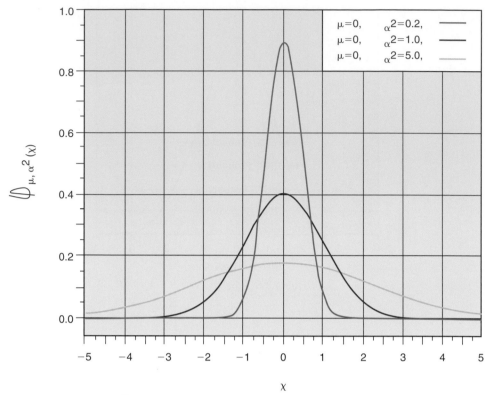

Figure 2-6 Standard deviations and predictability.

Whether we are working with clinical, financial, or administrative data, there are numerous instances when we might want to find the variance of an observation from the mean. For example, we might want to set up a frequency distribution for a sample of patients' lengths of stay (Figure 2-7).

In this set, we have a mean LOS of about 4 days. Now let us imagine we have a physician whose patient's ALOS is 7, varying 3 days longer than the average. If the standard deviation of ALOS for these patients is 1.66, then an ALOS of 7 is nearly 2 standard deviations from the mean $(4 + 1.66\,\sigma + 1.66\,\sigma = 7.32)$. That means this physician's ALOS is higher than 96% of all others.

LOS Length of stay.

ALOS Average length of stay.

	A	B	C	D	E	F	G	H	I	J	K
1											
2											
3											
4	DATA:										
5	Length of stay of 250 patients discharged in April, 2012										
6											
7	1	2	3	3	3	4	4	5	5	6	
8	1	2	3	3	3	4	4	5	5	6	
9	1	2	3	3	4	4	4	5	5	6	
10	1	2	3	3	4	4	4	5	5	6	
11	1	3	3	3	4	4	4	5	5	6	
12	1	3	3	3	4	4	4	5	5	6	
13	1	3	3	4	4	4	4	5	5	6	
14	1	3	3	4	4	4	4	5	5	6	
15	1	3	3	4	4	4	4	5	5	6	
16	2	3	3	4	4	4	4	5	5	6	
17	2	3	3	4	4	4	5	5	5	6	
18	2	3	3	4	4	4	5	5	5	6	
19	2	3	3	4	4	4	5	5	5	7	
20	2	3	3	4	4	4	5	5	5	7	
21	2	3	3	4	4	4	5	5	5	7	
22	2	3	3	4	4	4	5	5	5	7	
23	2	3	3	4	4	4	5	5	6	7	
24	2	3	3	4	4	4	5	5	6	7	
25	2	3	3	4	4	4	5	5	6	8	
26	2	3	3	4	4	4	5	5	6	8	
27	2	3	3	4	4	4	5	5	6	8	
28	2	3	3	4	4	4	5	5	6	8	
29	2	3	3	4	4	4	5	5	6	10	
30	2	3	3	4	4	4	5	5	6	12	
31	2	3	3	4	4	4	5	5	6	15	
32											
33	Mean = Total of all LOS / Number of patients										
34	=SUM(A7:J31)/250										
35	OR										
36	=AVERAGE(A7:J31)										
37	Mean = 4.144										
38											
39											
40	=STDEVP(A7:J31)										
41	Standard Deviation = 1.66										
42											
43											
44											
45											

LOS	Frequency	% of total patients
1	9	3.6%
2	20	8.0%
3	54	21.6%
4	77	30.8%
5	56	22.4%
6	21	8.4%
7	6	2.4%
8	4	1.6%
9	0	0.0%
10	1	0.4%
12	1	0.4%
15	1	0.4%
	0	
Total Patients	250	

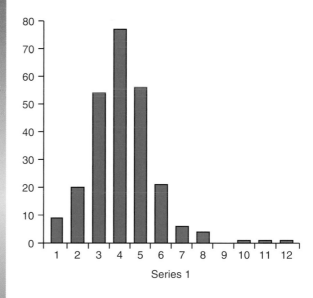

Figure 2-7 A frequency distribution for LOS.

REVIEW QUESTIONS

1. Convert the following improper fractions to mixed number fractions:

   a. $\dfrac{18}{8}$

   b. $\dfrac{21}{2}$

   c. $\dfrac{14}{12}$

2. Reduce the fractions below to their simplest form.

   a. $\dfrac{33}{66}$

   b. $\dfrac{5}{100}$

   c. $\dfrac{750}{1000}$

3. Add or subtract the following fractions. Report your answers in simple fractions.

   a. $\dfrac{1}{12} + \dfrac{7}{12}$

   b. $\dfrac{1}{8} - \dfrac{2}{3}$

   c. $4\dfrac{1}{2} - 3\dfrac{1}{5}$

4. Convert the following fractions to decimals:

   a. $\dfrac{1}{8}$

   b. $\dfrac{1}{22}$

   c. $\dfrac{14}{12}$

5. Round each decimal to the tenths place. Then round each to the hundredths place.

   a. 0.09513999
   b. 0.551001
   c. 22.7399
   d. 1.1733

6. Convert each percentage to decimal form, or vice versa.

    a. 55%
    b. 17%
    c. 1156%
    d. 0.034
    e. 0.78
    f. 1.11

7. The college has a 97% placement rate for its new graduates. If there are 111 students in this year's class, how many will find jobs?

8. Convert 25 mg to grams.

9. A baby weighs 8 lbs. 1 oz at birth. How many grams does she weigh?

10. To mix a certain medicine, you add one capful to every 8 ounces of water. How many capfuls do you need to make 64 ounces?

11. Your department has budgeted for three sets of references for every five coders. Recently, a reorganization moved all of the coding to your hospital, and now there are 25 coders. How many sets of references will you need?

12. What does calculating the mean tell you? What are its advantages and disadvantages?

13. The nursing home has 50 male patients and 86 female patients. What is the absolute frequency at the nursing home? What is the relative frequency of males? Of females? What is the ratio of men to women in its simplest form?

14. While looking at salaries of physician's assistants (PAs) in the health system, you find a range from a low of $85,000 to a high of $160,000. How many classes would you have if you broke them into class widths of $5000? What about widths of $20,000?

15. Fifty patients were treated at the free clinic last week. Their ages are listed from youngest to oldest: 14, 15, 15, 16, 16, 17, 17, 17, 17, 18, 18, 18, 19, 19, 19, 19, 19, 19, 20, 20, 20, 21, 21, 21, 22, 22, 24, 24, 24, 25, 26, 26, 26, 27, 28, 30, 31, 32, 36, 40, 41, 41, 47, 52, 52, 59, 59, 60, 65, 72.

    a. What is the mean age?
    b. What is the median?
    c. What is the mode?
    d. What is the range?
    e. Calculate the variance of the ages listed from a frequency distribution.
    f. Calculate the variance of the ages from a frequency distribution with class limits of 14 to 35, and a standard deviation with a class interval of 1.

CHAPTER

DATA PRESENTATION

CHAPTER OUTLINE

TABLES
    Design, Components, and Rules
        Table Construction: Simple or
            Complex?
        Formatting Tables
        Tools for Table Creation

GRAPHS AND CHARTS
    Line Graphs
    Scatter Diagrams
    Bar Charts and Bar Graphs
    Histograms

Pie Charts
Pictograms
REVIEW QUESTIONS

KEY TERMS

bar chart
contingency table
cross-tabulation
frequency table

histogram
line graph
pictogram
pivot table

precision
scatter diagram
x-axis
y-axis

LEARNING OBJECTIVES

At the end of the chapter, you should be able to do the following:
1. Construct a variety of tables using the guidelines given.
2. Critique samples of tables to determine missing or faulty elements.
3. Construct and interpret pie charts, line graphs, bar charts, pictograms, scatter diagrams, and histograms.
4. Give examples of how each of the graphic displays is best used.
5. Critique samples of charts and graphs to determine missing or faulty elements.

Once you collect the data needed and perform calculations to determine the information requested, you will need to arrange the resulting information into a format that displays those findings. The format choices are a written report, a table, and/or a graph. Depending on the request, you may want to do one, two, or all of the above. This chapter will help you decide which format(s) to use, which is best suited for the information you want to provide, and how to create each of them. By format, you will be exposed to the vocabulary and rules that are necessary to build useful, intelligent vehicles to deliver your work.

BRIEF CASE

WORKING WITH OTHERS

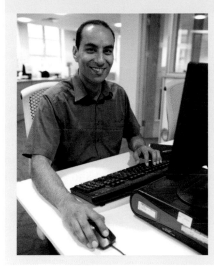

Things are a bit different at the office today—Sasha is excited to have a visitor! One of Sasha's favorite former instructors arranged an internship with a student, Prasad, who is shadowing Sasha for a few hours a day this week to gain some valuable on-the-job experience.

Calculating statistics is an obvious job requirement for a data analyst, and presenting the findings in a visual, easily accessible format is yet another. Adding well-chosen visuals to any presentation usually helps to get the point across much more easily, and the use of visuals in statistics is no exception.

Take a look at the following examples that are the results of an analysis of the numbers of discharged patients at a hospital during a particular time period. Your administrator asks you for data trends in overall discharges. Compare the following: one is a brief statement of the findings, the second is in tabular format, and the final is a line graph of the same.

① *"The patient discharges for the first four months of 2015 (January – April) showed a continual increase, starting with 467 in January and ending with 1598 in April."*

②

Patient Discharge Totals: January - April 2015	
Month	Discharges
January	467
February	802
March	1123
April	1598
Total	3990

③

Patient discharge totals: January-April 2015

—— Patient discharge totals: January-April 2015

Which of the three is your eye drawn to? Which communicates the findings in the quickest manner? What is happening with patient discharges from January to April? Can you see advantages and disadvantages of each of the formats (an actual statement of the conclusion in one, more detail in another, a quicker impression in yet another)? Note that if the question was different (*what are the actual numbers by month?*), you might choose a different answer. You will need to ask yourself some questions to choose the best means of data presentation. Do you need a summary or detailed findings? Are you showing a trend? A proportion? Keep your choices focused on what information you need to impart.

TABLES

Tax tables, multiplication tables, and tables of nutritional information are probably familiar to most of us. All consist of numerical information that is organized into rows and columns to facilitate reference to the data within. Well-constructed tables consist of a number of components that allow the information within to be understood without reference to any other sources. For example, the nutritional information table for your favorite cookies gives you the serving size, the number of servings in the package, the number of calories, calories from fat, the weight (in grams), and percent of Daily Value for several different attributes of the cookies. The entire table is self-contained, so you can find all of the nutritional information that has been measured and reported all in one neat tabular package. This table is an answer to the question, *what is the nutritional information regarding my favorite cookies?* (Figure 3-1)

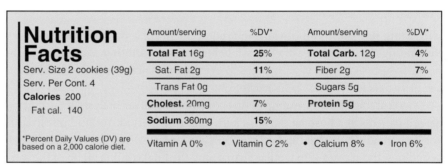

Figure 3-1 Nutritional value for your favorite cookies.

Stat Tip ··

An important step in the process of using statistics is the application of one's findings. Although these cookies are a good source of calcium, should the reader assume that they should become a dietary staple? Think back to the data pyramid we discussed in Chapter 1. While this table provides *information* regarding dietary choices, the information needs to be used in context to provide the *intelligence* required to make a decision as to how it should be used.

Design, Components, and Rules

Let us look at the important components and design considerations for constructing a table regarding health care data. Figure 3-2 shows the name of each of the design

Table Number. *Table Title.*		
Stub Head	**Box head**	
	Column head	Column head
Stub	Cell	Cell
Stub	Cell	Cell
Stub	Cell	Cell
Stub	Cell	Cell*
*Note: All the cells together are called a body.		

Table 1. *Discharges by month for St. Barnabas, January-April 2015*		
Month	**Discharges**	
	Men	Women
Jan	200	267
Feb	402	400
March	466	657
April	707	891*
*Note: This figure follows the opening of the new Sarah Platt Maternity Wing.		

Figure 3-2 Parts of a table.

components, along with a sample table on the right. While tables vary in complexity, virtually all tables will include the following elements:

Table Number

The table number is used to keep your displays organized. This is a useful feature for using tables that display the information in different configurations. For example, Table 1 may be a simple display of patient discharges by month, while Table 2 uses the same data, but breaks it down by discharges by service.

Title

The title of a table needs to give a quick and complete snapshot of the data within. As an easy memory device, you could consider answering all but one of the who, what, when, where, and why questions:
- Who is the data describing (e.g., type II diabetic patients, physicians)?
- What are the statistics that have calculated (e.g., percentages, proportions, averages)?
- When is the time period that is being examined (e.g., year, quarter, week)?
- Where do the data come from (e.g., hospital, physician practice, clinic)?
- Why? (There is no need to answer this one—because it is your job!)

Table Shell

Overall, you need to think of the general structure of the table. This is called the table shell. A well-constructed shell will allow you to place the data into predefined categories. The shell consists of the columns and rows that contain the data.

Box Head and Stubs

The box head or column header tells the reader what type of data is displayed in the columns, while the stub header does the same for the rows. While the column header is at the top of the table, the stub header is in the most left-hand column.

Box Heads

Column titles or captions name the individual columns, while stubs name the individual rows.

Cells

The intersection of a column and a row is referred to as a cell. In our sample table, you can see that the intersection of the number of women who were discharged and the month of January is the number 267. The meaning of this cell would be that there were 267 women discharged during the month of January alone.

Tables commonly contain more information than what was included in this sample. Added columns or rows may be used to describe totals or percentages to allow for some summary data regarding the categories within. They simply need to be labeled with stubs or box heads so that the reader knows what is contained in each. Footnotes or notes are any additional explanations for elements of the table or anything that is not displayed within the body of the table or the source explanation. An example might be an asterisk that appears next to the month of April that notes the addition of a new service for the hospital, which could help to explain that steep increase.

Finally, the source of your data tells the reader the origin of the data and allows him or her to reproduce the study using the same data if necessary or desired.

Table Construction: Simple or Complex?

Sometimes your table is as simple as our first example. Here, you are displaying the variation of one dependent variable (number of patient discharges) by the independent variable (month). You have one column header (patient discharges) and one stub header (months). You might ask, does it matter which is the column header and which is the stub header? No, it does not. It is a matter of preference as to which you think is best for your purposes.

What if that first table triggered a request for more detail? Say, for example, you are asked to not only report the total discharges, but you also need to report a breakdown by patient gender for each of those totals. Here, your column header would remain patient discharge totals, but underneath there would be two columns: one for male, and one for female. This allows you to compare the additional relationship of patient discharge by gender per month. How would this look? What if we needed a further breakdown to include the analysis of discharges by month, gender, and race? Figure 3-3 shows how we might arrange our simple table to accommodate the additional data.

Remember, think of what are you trying to convey. Your table will change depending on how many different items you measure. While one-variable tables are simple and easy to construct, two-variable tables (like the one mentioned above with discharges by gender and month) are referred to as **contingency tables** or **cross-tabulations**. As we will discover in later chapters, contingency tables will be important when we need to calculate inferential statistics from a sample of population data. Another consideration when constructing tables is awareness of the type of data that is appearing: is it qualitative, like gender or ICD-10 codes? Or is the data quantitative and able to be summed? Is the data discrete or continuous? Taking a minute to identify these now will reinforce your awareness for inferential statistics that may need to be calculated later.

Frequency tables (introduced in Chapter 2) are obvious displays of data that show how many of a category appears for each class interval. The columns include not only the totals, but also may include a cumulative (total) frequency column, a percentage frequency column, and a percentage of cumulative frequency column. Table 3-1 is a frequency table showing the distribution of grades received by students in a course. Remember that all of your data needs to fit into one—and only one—of your categories. That means that your categories need to be exhaustive (all the data you have fits into all the categories you have) and mutually exclusive (no piece of data could fit into more than one category). On the other hand, none of your cells should be empty. If there are no observations for a particular frequency or cell, then place a 0, a dash, or an N/A in it. (For example, a table showing top procedures by gender at a particular hospital would list N/A for total hysterectomies reported in the "Male" column.)

TAKE AWAY ●⋯⋯⋯

Health data analysts will need to be proficient at not only constructing data displays, but also at reading the information presented within them.

◉ **Contingency table** A table with two variables; also called a cross-tabulation.

◉ **Cross-tabulation** A table with two variables; also called a contingency table.

◉ **Frequency table** A tabular display showing how often an observation appears in each class of a frequency distribution.

Table 1. *Discharges by Month with Gender and Race Totals for St. Barnabas, January-April 2015*

| Month | Discharges | | | | | | Discharge Totals |
| | Male | | | Female | | | |
	White	NonWhite	Total	White	NonWhite	Total	White/Non White Totals
January	121	79	200	145	122	267	467
February	200	202	402	190	210	400	802
March	266	200	466	300	357	657	1123
April	350	357	707	500	391	891	1598
Totals	**937**	**838**	**1775**	**1135**	**1080**	**2215**	**3990**

Figure 3-3 Adding columns to show more specific data.

TABLE 3-1

A FREQUENCY TABLE

		COURSE GRADES				
CLASS (GRADE)	CLASS INTERVAL (GRADE RANGE)	VALUES	FREQUENCY (F)	CUMULATIVE FREQUENCY (CF)	PERCENTAGE FREQUENCY (%F)	PERCENTAGE OF CUMULATIVE FREQUENCY (%CF)
A	90-100	90, 90, 93, 97, 100	5	5	21.7%	21.7%
B	80-89	81, 83, 85, 85, 86, 88, 88, 89	8	13	34.8%	56.5%
C	70-79	70, 71, 73, 75, 75, 78, 78, 79	8	21	34.8%	91.3%
D	60-69	62	1	22	4.3%	95.6%
F	0-59	49	1	23	4.3%	99.9%

Precision The significant figures, or the number of digits to the right of a decimal.

Formatting Tables

The table number and title may be centered or left justified. The headings for the columns and rows can also be centered, left justified, or right justified. Cells should be left justified and the **precision** (the significant figures, or the number of digits for decimal places) should be the same for any decimals used.

BRIEF CASE

CHECKING YOUR WORK

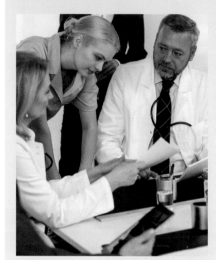

Sasha's manager asks for some information about how often the hospital treats patients with Type 1 diabetes by age for a meeting this afternoon with physicians who have privileges at the facility. Sasha gives Prasad data for the past six months and asks him to create a frequency table for use in the presentation. After lunch, Prasad puts together the table below.

TABLE 1. TREATMENT OF TYPE 1 DIABETES

AGE RANGE	F	CF	%F	%CF
91-100				100%
81-90	1	125	8.0	100%
71-80	3	124	2.4	99.2%
61-70	3	121	2.4	96.8%
51-60	7	118	5.6	94.4%
41-50	3	111	2.4	88.8%
31-40	4	108	3.2	86.4%
20-29	4	104	3.2	83.2%
11-20	50	100	40	80%
0-10	50	50	40	40%

How does Prasad's table look? Sasha remembered some of the mistakes she made when she was a student, and she was careful to check the table. What errors do you see?

Tools for Table Creation

Microsoft Excel and other spreadsheet applications contain very powerful tools for the data analyst. Formatting tables is made simple, with the ability to justify or center your title, box headers, stubs, and data; you can create custom borders, shade specific cells, or choose from hundreds of preformatted table designs. Not only does Excel make entering your data and designing your table an easier task, it can sort, count, and sum your data, and it provides a host of other statistical tools. As we will explore soon, it can even create graphs and charts to display your data visually.

Pivot table An Excel tool that extracts data from a large table into a smaller table.

One feature that data analysts use frequently to summarize the data in a lengthy table is called a pivot table. A **pivot table** works by automatically extracting the information you want to see and summarizing the information in a smaller, separate table. Figure 3-4 shows two different tables automatically extracted from a larger table using Excel's Pivot Table function.

Physician ID	ICD-10	Procedure	Gender	Year	Count
1897417386	0SR9	Hip Joint, Right	Male	2016	3
1897417386	0SRB	Hip Joint, Left	Male	2016	2
1897417386	0SR9	Hip Joint, Right	Female	2016	5
1897417386	0SRB	Hip Joint, Left	Female	2016	4
1897417386	0SRA	Hip Joint, Acetabular Surface, Right	Male	2016	2
1897417386	0SRE	Hip Joint, Acetabular Surface, Left	Male	2016	1
1897417386	0SRA	Hip Joint, Acetabular Surface, Right	Female	2016	3
1897417386	0SRE	Hip Joint, Acetabular Surface, Left	Female	2016	5
1897417386	0SRR	Hip Joint, Femoral Surface, Right	Male	2016	1
1897417386	0SRS	Hip Joint, Femoral Surface, Left	Male	2016	2
1897417386	0SRR	Hip Joint, Femoral Surface, Right	Female	2016	3
1897417386	0SRS	Hip Joint, Femoral Surface, Left	Female	2016	4
1897417386	0SR9	Hip Joint, Right	Male	2015	2
1897417386	0SRB	Hip Joint, Left	Male	2015	1
1897417386	0SR9	Hip Joint, Right	Female	2015	4
1897417386	0SRB	Hip Joint, Left	Female	2015	3
1897417386	0SRA	Hip Joint, Acetabular Surface, Right	Male	2015	1
1897417386	0SRA	Hip Joint, Acetabular Surface, Right	Female	2015	2
1897417386	0SRE	Hip Joint, Acetabular Surface, Left	Female	2015	4
1897417386	0SRS	Hip Joint, Femoral Surface, Left	Male	2015	1
1897417386	0SRR	Hip Joint, Femoral Surface, Right	Female	2015	2
1897417386	0SRS	Hip Joint, Femoral Surface, Left	Female	2015	3

Sum of Count by Year			
ICD-10	2015	2016	Grand Total
0SR9	6	8	14
0SRA	3	5	8
0SRB	4	6	10
0SRE	4	6	10
0SRR	2	4	6
0SRS	4	6	10
Grand Total	23	35	58

Sum of Count by Gender			
ICD-10	Female	Male	Grand Total
0SR9	9	5	14
0SRA	5	3	8
0SRB	7	3	10
0SRE	9	1	10
0SRR	5	1	6
0SRS	7	3	10
Grand Total	42	16	58

Figure 3-4 Pivot tables automatically extract information from a larger table into smaller ones.

EXERCISE 3-1

1. Another name for a box head is a _____, which tells the reader what type of data is displayed in the columns.

2. What type of table shows how many of a category appears for each class interval?

3. Explain how pivot tables make it easier to see relationships in a set of data.

GRAPHS AND CHARTS

Charts and graphs are visual impressions of summarized data. While they leave out the specifics of the actual findings, they provide a swift understanding of the results. There are a number of options, and each will have its advantages, disadvantages, and best uses (see Table 3-2). Excel provides a number of options for graphic presentation of its data. Its Chart Wizard creates quickly constructed visuals that can then be exported to Microsoft Word or PowerPoint for your reporting needs. The individual graph or chart still needs to be numbered and titled, and sources and any footnotes are also required.

Line Graphs

Line graphs A graphical display of data connecting coordinates with a line, useful for showing trends over time.

X-axis The horizontal (left-to-right) axis.

Y-axis The vertical axis, showing the frequency of the dependent variable.

Line graphs are best used to illustrate trends in the frequency of data. The data is laid out on a graph with an *x-axis* and a *y-axis*. The **x-axis** (the horizontal one) is used to place the independent variables, while the **y-axis** is used to record the frequency of the dependent variable. The location of the data point that is to be plotted is called a *coordinate*, and it is named for its position on the x and y axes (x, y). Figure 3-5 shows the components of a line graph.

For example, perhaps you are asked to graph the frequency of those patient discharges by month (Figure 3-6). Your horizontal axis (the y-axis) shows the months, while the vertical axis (the x-axis) records the frequency of discharges. A line is used to connect the data points. This is a good way to be able to see trends of increase, decrease, or no change in your data, especially over time. The advantages of a line graph are that it provides a quick picture of the trend, and it is easy to graph. On the other hand, unless a coordinate is labeled, exact data values may not be available. And, most importantly, unless one starts the graph with the origins of the axes at (0, 0), an exaggerated

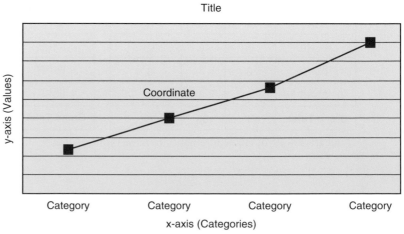

Figure 3-5 Components of a line graph.

result can be visualized. For example, the first graph of discharges from January to April in Figure 3-6 has an increase from 467 to 1598 discharges. If we changed the scale on the y-axis from starting at 0 to starting at 400 and ending at 1600, you can see that our reported increase appears to be much more dramatic.

If the scale does not start at zero (or if the analyst wants to show that the scale is not continuous from zero), a tear mark or break is used to signify an interruption in a continuous, consistent scale from zero. Figure 3-7 is a line graph that shows thousands of admissions, ranging from 12,000 to 14,000 throughout a 10-year period. The change is small, so it would seem that plotting it on a zero scale gives a very slight slope. A tear mark would allow the line to be more centrally located in the graph and still accurately present the information.

Scatter Diagrams

Another type of chart that uses coordinates is a scatter diagram (also called a scatter plot or X-Y plot). **Scatter diagrams** help visualize suspected cause and effect relationships between independent and dependent variables. For example, a coding supervisor has been trying to manage the workload of an increase in the number of charts that need to be coded from a recent corresponding increase in admissions. While her coders have been getting the charts coded, she has also seen the percentage of miscoded charts increase. She suspects that it might be from the charts coded with overtime hours. In this case, the independent variable is the overtime hour, and the dependent

○ **Scatter diagram** A type of chart that uses coordinates to help visualize suspected cause and effect relationships between independent and dependent variables.

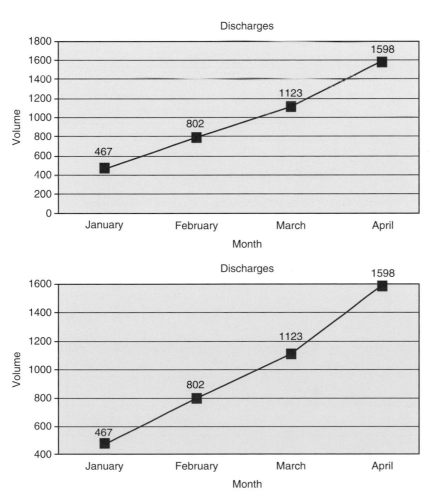

Figure 3-6 Line graph showing discharges by month for St. Barnabas, January to April, 2015.

variable is the number of errors. To take a look at the problem, she collects the errors that occurred by coder and assigns them to the number of overtime hours. Her table is as follows:

	ERRORS		
Coder	**Hour 1**	**Hour 2**	**Hour 3**
Aisha	5	7	8
Brittnee	8	13	12
Carol	7	9	14
Delilah	5	9	10
Edie	4	5	8
Totals	29	43	52

Once the coding supervisor had her table set up, she used Excel to plot the data (Figure 3-8), and she could see that there was a trend. The more overtime hours

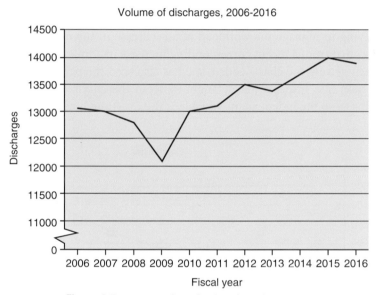

Figure 3-7 Line graph with a break in the x-axis.

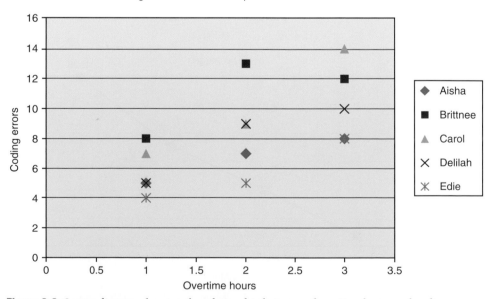

Figure 3-8 Scatter diagram showing the relationship between of overtime hours and coding errors.

that were logged by her staff, the more errors occurred. As a result, she weighed the cost of making errors and then correcting them versus the cost of hiring temporary coders.

Bar Charts and Bar Graphs

Bar charts and **bar graphs** also use an x- and y-axis. The frequencies represented, however, are bars or columns instead of a coordinate of the two axes. Bar charts are an excellent choice for representing categorical or nominal data, like gender, race, marital status, and zip code, where the bars do not touch because the data is not continuous. (Remember that you cannot perform mathematical calculations on categorical data; no one is 1.25 married.) While the main disadvantage of a bar chart is that it cannot use continuous data, they are, however, easy to construct, use x and y axes like the line graphs, and can be modified to show more detailed results by using stacked bars. Excel allows you to decide if you want to present the bars vertically (they refer to it as a column chart) or horizontally (called a bar chart). Figure 3-9 shows patient discharges by ethnicity (a categorical value) in both types of bar graph.

Histograms

Histograms are graphic displays of frequency distributions. The rectangles formed by the connection of the heights of the frequencies of the class intervals form bars that touch. Histograms are used to display continuous data that has been organized into a series of intervals. The advantage of histograms is in its display of the frequency of continuous data. That said, they are not useful for displaying data that is of a discrete nature. The area within each of the class interval rectangles is the same as the percentage of each interval to the total number of scores under study. A histogram (and the data used to construct it) is shown in Figure 3-10.

Pie Charts

Pie charts present data categories in percentages of a whole. They are best used to show comparisons of the proportions of categories to each other. For example, a discharge disposition is a type of categorical (nominal) data, in that a patient cannot be transferred to home *and* to a hospice. A pie chart would be a great way to display how our patients left the hospital. Are most discharged to home? Were they transferred? Did they expire (die)? Did they leave against medical advice (AMA)? Figure 3-11 provides that information to the reader in a quick glance.

In pie charts, data needs to be converted from the actual subtotals to percentages, then placed in ascending or descending order. When constructing a pie chart, keep in mind the number of categories in your data; when too many categories are used, pie charts can be difficult to read, and their impact is diminished.

Bar graph A graphical display of data in which the values of variables are represented by the height or length of lines or rectangles; also called a bar chart.

Bar chart A graphical display of data in which the values of variables are represented by the height or length of lines or rectangles; also called a bar graph.

Histograms Graphic displays of frequency distributions.

Pie Chart A graphical presentation of data showing data categories as percentages of a whole.

AMA Against medical advice.

MATH REVIEW

A proportion is the relationship between one part and the whole, or one part and another part.

Stat Tip

In a pie chart, all the slices will always add up to 100%.

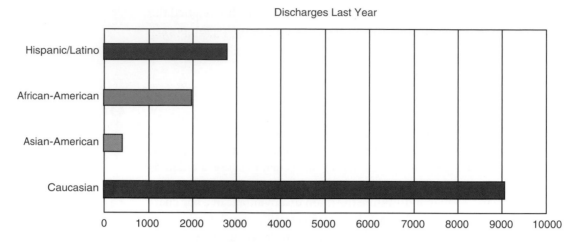

Ethnicity	Discharges Last Year
Caucasian	9054
Asian-American	421
African-American	1978
Hispanic/Latino	2798

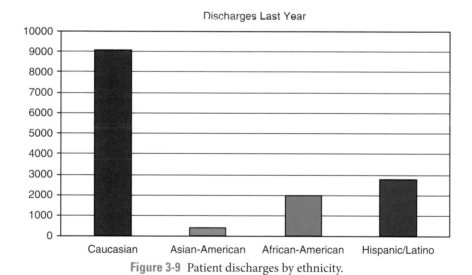

Figure 3-9 Patient discharges by ethnicity.

Histogram Showing the Distribution of Class Grades

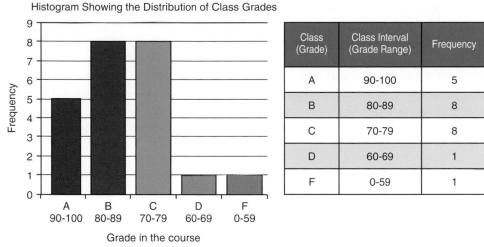

Class (Grade)	Class Interval (Grade Range)	Frequency
A	90-100	5
B	80-89	8
C	70-79	8
D	60-69	1
F	0-59	1

Figure 3-10 Histogram showing the distribution of class grades.

Discharge Disposition, 2015

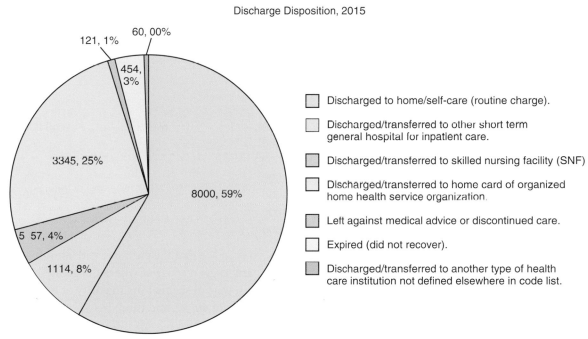

- Discharged to home/self-care (routine charge).
- Discharged/transferred to other short term general hospital for inpatient care.
- Discharged/transferred to skilled nursing facility (SNF)
- Discharged/transferred to home card of organized home health service organization.
- Left against medical advice or discontinued care.
- Expired (did not recover).
- Discharged/transferred to another type of health care institution not defined elsewhere in code list.

Figure 3-11 2015 Discharge disposition.

Virtually all data managers will create a pie chart using software (like Excel), but knowing how they are created will help you understand how they can and should be used. Let us look at an example of a good pie chart and a bad one. Say we wanted to show the incidence of peptic ulcer bleeding (PUB) among all patients, by age from 0 to 94. This disorder is very, very rare in children, but for the sake of illustration, let us create a pie chart using intervals of five years (i.e., 0–4, 5–9, 10–14, etc., Figure 3-12, A). In another pie chart, we will choose much wider intervals of 20 years (0–19, 20–39, 40–59, 60–79, > 80, displayed in Figure 3-12, B). Here is our data from the national database, arranged in the narrower and wider intervals.

PUB Peptic ulcer bleeding.

Ages (Class Intervals)	Incidence (Frequency)	Ages (Class Intervals)	Incidence (Frequency)
0-4	1	0-19	29
5-9	1		
10-14	7		
15-19	20		
20-24	1200	20-39	19,800
25-29	3600		
30-34	6000		
35-39	9000		
40-44	15,000	40-59	65,000
45-49	16,000		
50-54	16,000		
55-59	18,000		
60-64	18,000	60-79	60,000
65-69	15,000		
70-74	15,000		
75-79	12,000		
80-84	5000	>80	11,000
85-89	3000		
> 90	3000		

Looking at the illustrations, you can see that the pie chart with almost 20 intervals is very difficult to read. It is even hard to get a sense of where the greatest concentration of ages are. But with fewer intervals, we can see that the majority of individuals treated for this disorder are between the ages of 40-59, and those between 40 and 79 make up the vast majority of all cases.

TABLE 3-2

SUMMARY OF GRAPHS AND CHARTS

TYPE	DESCRIPTION	ILLUSTRATION	TYPES OF DATA	USES	ADVANTAGES	DISADVANTAGES	EXAMPLES OF USE
Table	Numerical material presented in tabular formata		All data types	Actual data results	More info than graphic displays Requires less work to create	Not as attractive or eye catching as a graph or chart Difficult to detect trends and patterns	Cancer stages, Nutritional information
Histogram	Shows the frequency of categories of continuous data		Continuous	To visualize the shape of the data	Shows the relationships of the data categories to each other	Only useful for continuous data	Weights, temperatures, salaries, square footage
Line graph	Shows trends in data, specifically over time		Continuous	To determine if there are increases, decreases, or no change in measures under observation	Provides a quick picture of the type of trend Easy to graph	Exact data values are not available	Frequency of discharges, census data, births, deaths, procedures
Scatter diagram	Shows actual data points that can be used to examine relationships		Continuous	To determine if there is a relationship between the two variables	Shows a trend in the data relationship Retains exact data values and sample size Shows minimum/maximum and outliers	Can be difficult to see trends in a large number of data points	Medicine and test results

Continued

TABLE 3-2

SUMMARY OF GRAPHS AND CHARTS—cont'd

Bar graph/ chart	Groupings of data into columns and rows		Categorical	Familiar, easy to read format Useful for comparing data within and outside of results (as long as scale remains the same)	Can only be used with categorical data	Display of gender, race, zip code, diagnoses, DRGs, Likert scale results
Pie chart	Representation of percentages of a whole. Useful for presenting proportions instead of actual quantities		All data types	Attractive and familiar Gives an immediate impression of relative size of category	No exact numerical data Hard to compare 2 data sets "Other" category can be a problem Total unknown unless specified Best for 3 to 7 categories Use only with discrete data	Comparison of patients of different races, gender, marital status, by medical/surgical service
Pictogram/ picto-graph	Uses icons to represent quantities/ units of data		Categorical	A catchy display of discrete data Easy to read Attractive Useful for displaying large volumes of data	Partial icons may be difficult to understand Size of icons can distort presentation of findings May appear to be not serious Icons require a key	Number of patients, materials, anything that can be represented by an icon.

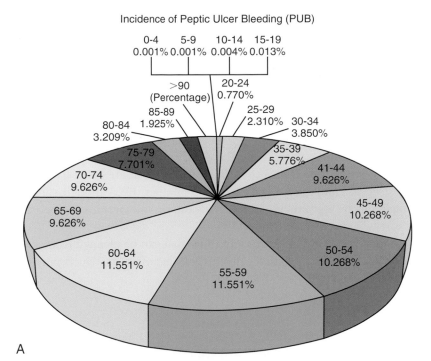

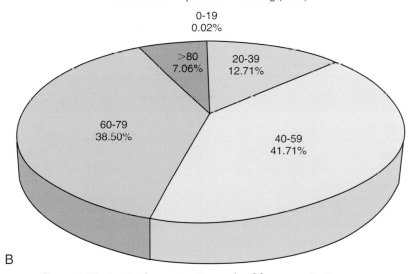

Figure 3-12 A, Pie chart using intervals of five years. **B,** 20 years.

Pictograms

○ **Pictogram** A graphical display using icons to represent numbers.

Pictograms (sometimes called pictographs) use icons instead of numbers to represent units of data. (Figure 3-13).

A pictogram, like any other data presentation method, has its advantages and disadvantages. (See Figure 3-14 for a pictogram showing the advantages and disadvantages of pictograms.) On one hand, pictograms are an incredibly engaging, attractive way to present data. They are useful in conveying a sense of large findings by using icons to represent units. On the other hand, the disadvantages include possible distortions of data, the need to round off data to fit into the units that are being used, and confusion when used to compare one pictogram to another. Even though sometimes the disadvantages of a pictogram outweigh the advantages, pictograms can be a clever and engaging way to communicate your findings.

Excel provides its own pictograms and those that can be gleaned from a search for free icons on the internet. Microsoft calls this feature SmartArt, which can be accessed from the "Insert" tab.

BRIEF CASE

USING GRAPHS

Sasha checks her email and sees one last request of the day. Prasad has been asking for an opportunity to work with graphing, so she gives him the accounts receivable table for three of their hospitals. She asks him to give her a stacked bar chart for each payer by hospital.

Payer	St. Barnabas	Happy Valley Community	Midtown General
Medicare	4600	5515	6540
Medicaid	1175	1487	1666
Blue Cross/Blue Shield	1254	1458	1631
Commercial Carriers	1056	1352	1502
Self-Pay	197	98	333
Indigent Care	336	333	248
Other Payers	197	155	64
Total	8815	10398	11984

What would this bar chart look like? Use the data in the table to create your own.

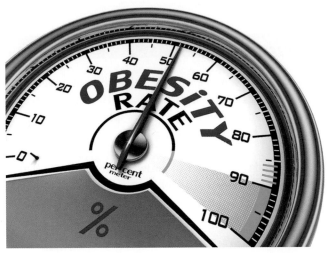

Figure 3-13 A pictogram using an image of a scale to present the obesity rate.

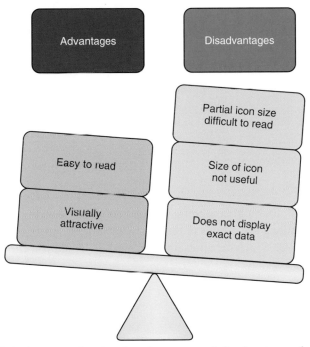

Figure 3-14 A pictogram showing the advantages and disadvantages of pictograms.

1. In January, 25 patients of Acme Home Health Nursing were Spanish speakers, while 75 spoke English. In February, there were 10 Spanish-speaking patients and 82 English speakers, and in March, 17 patients spoke Spanish and 90 spoke English. Present your data in a table with totals.

2. The free clinic counted the number of patients it treated who had no health insurance over the course of one year. The following table reflects their data. Present the information in both a stacked bar chart and a line graph.

Month	Male	Female
January	56	75
February	38	94
March	60	128
April	60	99
May	88	101
June	87	121
July	86	131
August	90	129
September	75	90
October	76	76
November	56	77
December	45	88

3. You are asked to build a graphic display of data showing the frequency of heart failure among age groups in the following ranges: 31-40, 41-50, 51-60, 61-70, 71-80, and 81-90. Which data presentation method would you choose (histogram)?

APPLICATIONS OF DESCRIPTIVE STATISTICS AND DATA ANALYSIS IN HEALTH CARE SETTINGS

ADMINISTRATIVE DATA

CHAPTER OUTLINE

KEY TERMS

average daily census
average length of stay (ALOS)
bassinet count
bed count
census

discharge days
encounter
inpatient service days (IPSDs)
leave of absence (LOA) day
length of stay (LOS)

observation bed
occupancy
swing bed

LEARNING OBJECTIVES

At the conclusion of this chapter, you should be able to do the following:

- Differentiate between inpatient and outpatient settings, listing examples of each.
- List the types of beds in an inpatient facility and calculate the bed count.

- Describe the inpatient census, inpatient service days, and how they are calculated.
- Calculate occupancy rates in a facility.
- Compute length of stay, average length of stay, leave of absence days, and bed turnover rate.

Health care is a business that takes place in a variety of settings, from walk-in clinics and physicians' offices to hospitals and nursing homes. While the services vary in intensity and expense, valuable statistics are collected in every setting to reflect the number of patients that were treated, their relative proportion to the facility's capacity, and how long the treatment lasts. All these statistics help the administrators and managers of these facilities determine how busy they are and what kinds of resources are being used, offering clues about what types services they should plan to provide for more efficient health care.

So what are we measuring? Beds, patients, and time. In essence, we are quantifying how many patients are being treated in our facility for a specified period of time; but we also have many different types of patients, different ways of counting time periods, and various ways of determining the available spots where the patients can stay. Because of this, we have standardized definitions for the way we measure services and some terminology about the different health care settings to cover.

BRIEF CASE

UNDERSTANDING THE FACILITY

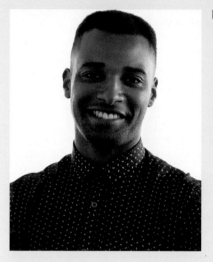

Michael has had the position of Health Care Data Technician at Diamonte Health for three years now, and each day brings new challenges and new rewards. Today, he opens his email to find a laundry list of work requests. The system administrator has apparently asked for comparison data between their three different hospitals regarding *utilization*, a measure of how much these hospitals' resources are being used. He will need to produce the statistics regarding *average daily census*, *occupancy*, and *average length of stay* (ALOS) for each of the hospitals over the prior year. The system administrator has also asked for a table and graph that summarizes the data for occupancy. Michael takes another sip of coffee and pulls out a pad of paper to make notes regarding what he will need for the task.

● **ALOS** Average length of stay.

● **CT** Computed tomography.

We can divide the people we treat into two kinds of patients: outpatients and inpatients. Outpatients are those we intend to care for within the same calendar day. A physician's office, for example, treats patients on an outpatient basis. Hopefully, if you go to a doctor's office or clinic, you do not expect to stay overnight. If you go to a radiology center to get a CT scan, you are treated as an outpatient. We call the health care settings that treat outpatients *ambulatory care facilities*, and in addition to doctor's offices and diagnostic services, like radiology and laboratory centers, other types of ambulatory care include same day surgery centers (also called ambulatory surgery centers) and emergency departments.

TAKE AWAY ●··········

Ambulatory care facilities treat outpatients, whose treatment is intended to occur within one calendar day.

Stat Tip ··································

The word ambulatory is from the Latin root *ambulo-*, which means *walking*. (If you are being treated on an ambulatory care or outpatient basis, we would expect you to walk out.)

"But wait," you say, "sometimes people go to the emergency department at the hospital and end up staying overnight, or even longer." You are, of course, correct. In the emergency department, patients arrive as outpatients, and many are treated for an illness or injury and go home. At other times, a physician will decide that a patient requires care for a longer period of time than the emergency department can provide. In these instances, the physician will write an *order to admit* an individual to the hospital as an inpatient. An inpatient is a person who will usually be treated overnight. Not all inpatients are admitted to a hospital through the emergency department, but all inpatient care requires a physician's order.

Some hospitals are classified as *acute care facilities*. The word *acute* means sudden or severe, and so acute care facilities are meant to handle inpatients whose illness or injury arises swiftly or severely. By definition, an acute care facility is a health care setting in which we expect to treat inpatients over an average of 30 days or less—and quite often, much less than that. But acute care facilities are not the only place we treat inpatients. Long-term care (LTC) facilities specialize in treating inpatients who tend to stay, on average, 30 days or more. A nursing home is one type of LTC facility—its patients need constant care for a time period much longer than 30 days. A skilled nursing facility (SNF) is another example: inpatients at SNFs, who usually have chronic, incurable illnesses, receive a range of nursing and auxiliary health care services. Other inpatient settings include behavioral health facilities, treating mental health disorders, and rehabilitation facilities, offering a variety of specific therapies as a result of illness or injury. Again, in all these settings, a doctor's order is required for an inpatient admission, though many offer outpatient services as well. Table 4-1 summarizes the health care settings treating inpatients and outpatients.

TAKE AWAY ●·········

A physician writes an order for an individual to be admitted as an inpatient, meaning he or she is intended to be treated overnight.

● **LTC**   Long-term care.

● **SNF**   Skilled nursing facility.

TABLE 4-1

TYPES OF HEALTH CARE SETTINGS

SETTING	TYPE OF CARE	DESCRIPTION
Acute care facility	Inpatient	A health care setting in which patients have an average stay of 30 days or less and that has an emergency department, operating suite, and clinical departments to handle a broad range of treatments.
Skilled nursing facility	Inpatient	A long-term care facility providing a range of nursing and other health care services to patients who require continuous care, typically those with a chronic illness.
Nursing home	Inpatient	A facility for older adults and individuals with physical disabilities who need constant care but at a lesser level than those in an skilled nursing facility.
Rehabilitation facility	Inpatient and outpatient	Offers care to patients who need specific therapies as a result of an illness or injury (e.g., respiratory failure, cerebrovascular accidents, joint replacement therapy).
Behavioral health facility	Inpatient and outpatient	Focuses on the treatment of psychiatric conditions.
Hospice	Inpatient and outpatient (home care)	Palliative health care services traditionally rendered to the terminally ill, their families, and their friends.
Physician's office or clinic	Outpatient	Ambulatory care in which the primary provider is the physician.
Ambulatory surgery center (same day surgery)	Outpatient	Surgical procedures performed on an outpatient basis; the patient returns home after the surgery is performed.
Emergency department	Outpatient	A part of a hospital with the equipment and staff to treat patients who require immediate care.
Diagnostic facility (radiology/ laboratory services)	Outpatient	Provides imaging (X-rays, CT scans, MRIs) and lab work (blood tests, urinalysis).
Home health care	Outpatient	Patients receive health care services in their residences.

The standard statistics to measure inpatient services are patient census, occupancy, and length of stay. In outpatient settings, we measure by *encounters* or *visits*. Several other statistics measure variations on these themes, each of which give us a different insight on the amount of patients we treat and how long it takes to treat them; they will be discussed as the chapter progresses.

OUTPATIENT STATISTICS

Patient Encounters

Encounter A patient's interaction with a health care provider to receive services; a unit of measure for the volume of ambulatory care services provided.

A patient **encounter** (also called a patient visit) is the scheduled face-to-face meeting of a patient and a health care provider for reasons of medical care (Figure 4-1). Patient encounters occur in outpatient facilities, like physicians' offices, ambulatory surgery centers, and hospital emergency departments. Measured in simple whole numbers, calculations on encounter data compare the patient volume by physician, by specialty, and/or by a specific time period.

A same day surgery center, for example, can offer a number of surgical services performed by several different surgeons. A single facility might provide plastic or reconstructive surgery, oral/dental surgery, podiatry, orthopedic surgery, colorectal surgery, and more. The practice manager might be interested in the number of visits each of the physicians in his/her practice is seeing per week. Those visits are most often reported as averages or medians with their accompanying ranges.

Remember that keeping track of the patient volume is one of many indicators of the health of a physician practice. While one physician may see the largest numbers of patients

MATH REVIEW

Means and medians tell us how often a value *usually* occurs. To find the mean (or average), sum the values and divide by the total number of observations. When we calculate the median, we are looking midpoint of a distribution. We arrange the scores from low to high or high to low and find the score that lies in the middle of the distribution.

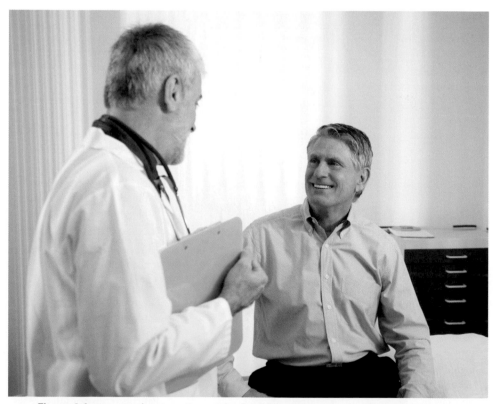

Figure 4-1 A patient's interaction with a health care provider is called an encounter.

over time, more data is necessary to determine whether this is a good thing or a bad thing financially—we need compare the reimbursement for those patients. A given physician may see the most patients, but because the reimbursement rate is so low, the practice makes very little profit from the effort. To have a viable business, the payment for services needs to be received in a timely manner and be enough to pay for its overhead costs.

EXERCISE 4-1
Outpatient Calculations

The table below lists the visit counts over a 4-week period at a practice that employs five physicians. Fill in the blank columns and rows to determine the means and ranges for each physician and each week.

PHYSICIAN	VISIT TOTAL WK 1	VISIT TOTAL WK 2	VISIT TOTAL WK 3	VISIT TOTAL WK 4	PHYSICIAN VISIT AVG	4-WEEK RANGE
Andrews	32	41	26	27	____	____
Basile	14	19	22	45	____	____
Chambers	31	34	32	31	____	____
Dahl	25	8	16	25	____	____
Edwards	27	14	16	23	____	____
Totals	129	116	112	151	____	____
Weekly average	____	____	____	____	____	____
Weekly physician range	____	____	____	____	____	____

1. Which physician had the highest volume of patients this month? Who averaged the most encounters per week?

2. Which physician had the widest range of encounters this month? Who had the narrowest?

3. How much does Dr. Edward's average differentiate from the facility's mean?

INPATIENT STATISTICS

Acute care hospitals are the traditional setting for patients who require treatment in an overnight setting. Because this setting is overnight, the service units are measured in the bed count.

Beds and Bed Count

Hospitals vary greatly in size from small (fewer than 100 beds) to medium (100–399) to large (400+).[1] Hospitals have a number of licensed beds for patients that *could* be used. Each state allows its hospitals a specific number of licensed beds, based on the needs of the community it serves. You can think of licensed beds as the maximum number of beds a hospital is allowed to have, but the number of beds that are physically in a hospital may be much lower. That being said, of those beds that are physically available, an even lower number of them have the staffing necessary to treat the patients who would

---

[1] http://www.ahadataviewer.com/glossary/.

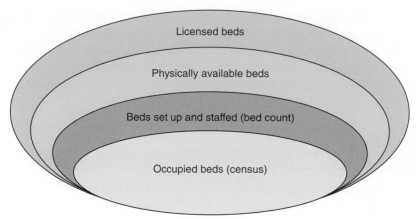

Figure 4-2 Types of beds in an inpatient facility. (Adapted from the *ESF 8 Resource Management's Definition of Bed Poll Terms* (https://esf8.dhh.la.gov/documentportal/Download/Public/Definitions%20of%20Bed%20Poll%20Terms.pdf) and from the AHRQ http://archive.ahrq.gov/research/havbed/definitions.htm.)

⊙ **Bed count** The actual number of beds that a hospital has staffed, equipped, and otherwise made available for occupancy by patients for each specific operating day.

fill them. In health care, we call this the **bed count**: the number of beds in the facility that are staffed and ready for patients, whether they are occupied or not. An even lower number of beds are actually occupied by patients. Figure 4-2 shows the relationship between licensed beds, those that are set up and staffed (the bed count), and the number of occupied beds, counted in a *census*.

Stat Tip ·······································

The bed count is sometimes called the *bed complement*, drawing from the word complement in the sense of complete, not the other compliment where nice things are said about them.

One bed set up for a patient for one 24-hour period, whether occupied or not, is measured as one *bed count day*. In short, the number of physical beds in the facility and bed count days are not the same. Where the beds are the potential for hospital usage, a bed count day is a measure of the usage of a hospital resource. Hospitals routinely sum bed count days over a period of time to determine how much of their resources are able to be used.

Types of Beds

The hospital does not confuse beds with bassinets: it would be inappropriate to place a newborn in an adult-sized bed, and impossible to put an adult in a bassinet. Inpatient beds are for use by adults and children, not newborn babies, so when it comes to counting how many adults and children the hospital can accommodate, we count those beds separately. Bassinets are used for the *newborn* population, and they are included in the **bassinet count**. An occupied bassinet or one that is ready for a newborn (also for the same 24-hour period) is considered to be one *bassinet count day*.

⊙ **Bassinet count** The actual number of bassinets that a hospital has staffed, equipped, and otherwise made available for occupancy by newborns for each specific operating day.

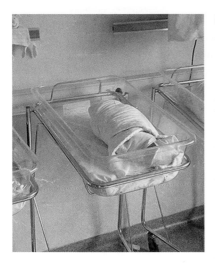

Some facilities also use *swing beds* for adults and children. Smaller hospitals may need to adjust the number of beds they have designated for shorter, acute care stays and those reserved for longer stays of more than 30 days. **Swing beds** are those that can have two different uses: either acute or LTC, depending on what is needed. They are used to provide the possibility of more skilled nursing care services for patients after acute care stays. To use swing beds, the hospital must meet a number of criteria, including Medicare participation and location in a rural area. Although the calculation of *swing bed days* are used to measure hospital utilization, they are also instrumental in the evaluation of costs when combined with the different types of reimbursements.

Beds can be temporary, too, set up and staffed in certain circumstances. During a natural disaster, for instance, disaster beds may be set up to accommodate the influx of patients. (Refer to Box 4-1 for a discussion of observation beds and the special calculations that can tell us about the quality of care patients are receiving.) Delivery room beds are those that are used temporarily for mothers who are giving birth. **Observation beds** are used for patients who need care that may extend overnight but do not yet merit an actual hospital admission. Beds such as these are considered temporary and are not included in the normal bed count.

Inpatient Census

Counting the patients who occupy those beds that are set up and staffed for use is the basis of a hospital's **census**: the number of patients who occupy those beds at a uniform time every day. A hospital's daily census is the number of "heads in bed," usually at midnight.

BOX 4-1	OBSERVATION STATUS

Patients may be in a type of limbo status, where they are in the hospital for one or more days, staying overnight, but are not formally admitted to the hospital. The National Health and Safety Network, a division of the CDC, directs that these days be counted as encounters (http://www.cdc.gov/nhsn/PDFs/PatientDay_SumData_Guide.pdf), and patients are given the designation of *observation status*. The reason for this type of care is to give the providers time to test and determine if the patient needs to be admitted or can be released to home. Observation status has become a topic in the discussion of measurement of readmission rates, or how often a patient returns to a facility for more treatment. Since facilities aim to keep their readmission rates low, providers may use observation status to determine whether a patient truly needs to be admitted to the hospital or not.

The AHRQ, an agency within the United States Department of Health and Human Services (HHS), uses a 30-day readmission rate formula as follows:

$$\frac{\text{The number of stays with at least one subsequent hospital stay within 30 days}}{\text{The total number of hospital stays between January and November}}$$

Source: http://hcupnet.ahrq.gov/HCUPnet.app/Methods-HCUPnet%20readmissions.pdf

Although census data is collected digitally at most hospitals, it is a good idea to be able to walk through how those numbers are collected and aggregated into a facility-wide census. Following through the example will also show you where the pitfalls are should you ever need to check and reconcile the results.

Designated hospital employees are assigned the responsibility of counting the number of patients filling the beds on their particular units at an agreed upon time across the facility. Each of the unit reports is summed into the total census for the hospital. Those numbers are aggregated for use as a reflection of the total number of adults, children, and newborns that are in the facility on any given day. We always calculate the adults and children census separately from the bassinet census.

Because patients may be transferred between units, the adherence of a facility to one facility-wide census taking time is important (always at midnight, for example). Otherwise, a patient could be counted twice (or not at all) as they move from one unit to another.

A patient admission is the formal acceptance of a patient to a health care facility for purposes of treatment. An admission requires a doctor's written order, though the admission of newborns to a hospital is traditionally through the act of being born in the hospital.

This sounds simple, though there are some situations to note. What happens, for instance, if a patient dies in the ambulance on the way to the hospital, is pronounced dead by the physician, and is placed in the morgue? A patient who arrives at the hospital dead on arrival (DOA) is **not** an admission. Patients who are not alive cannot be admitted to a hospital.

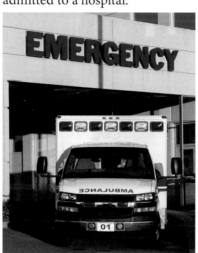

What about a baby born on the way to the hospital, in the parking lot, or even in the emergency room? These patients are considered "adult and children" admissions, as opposed to newborn admissions. And although they are provided care in a bassinet, they are not counted as occupying a bassinet. This is because the bassinet count is tailored to reflect the number of births the hospital can handle.

A patient discharge is the formal release of a patient from the hospital, again through the act of a doctor's written order. The patient's *disposition* is the manner of discharge from the hospital. The most common type of disposition is discharged to home, although others include leaving against medical advice (AMA), where a patient leaves against the consent of his/her physician, transfer between hospitals, and death.

In regard to the census, a patient being admitted to the hospital is an addition to the total, while a discharge is subtracted. An *inter* hospital transfer sends the patient to another facility altogether; this is a form of discharge, so it is always subtracted from the hospital total. An *intra*hospital transfer, where the patient is transferred between units within the same facility, is subtracted from the unit he/she came from and added to the unit he/she goes to.

Occasionally, a patient is admitted to the hospital and is subsequently discharged before the 24-hour period elapses. This situation (called admitted and discharged same day, or A&D) might occur when a patient is admitted and dies, is transferred, or decides to leave AMA. In this case, simply adding and subtracting the patient appears to have no effect on the census. Because the patient was there, and because health care personnel set up and staffed the bed, it would be unrealistic to "lose" the measure of a census day for this patient. For this reason, we add patients who were admitted and discharged the same day in a separate calculation to report total **inpatient service days (IPSDs)** that give us the daily inpatient census. An IPSD is a measure of the use of hospital services, representing the care provided to one inpatient during a 24-hour period. While the census shows how full the hospital is at one particular time during a day, the total IPSDs show how much work the hospital has done in that 24-hour period.

> **Inpatient service day (IPSD)** A measure of the use of hospital services representing the care provided to one inpatient during a 24-hour period.

Stat Tip

Some facilities call an IPSD a *census day*.

Let us take a look at a simple census on a surgical service within a hospital. The unit is set up and staffed with 24 beds. The hospital's census taking time is midnight. At midnight there are 20 patients occupying 20 of the 24 beds. This means that the midnight census is 20. During the next 24 hours, three more patients are admitted, while six of the patients are discharged. The following midnight, the census is 17 because $20 + 3 - 6 = 17$.

In a table format, those numbers would look like this:

HAPPY VALLEY HOSPITAL SURGICAL SERVICE: FEBRUARY 7, 2016

Adm/Disch	Census at Midnight	20
Admissions	+	3
Discharges	-	6
Patients at 11:59 p.m.	Total	17

But what if we had, in addition to the above, two patients who were A&D? Imagine that on the 7th, two patients were admitted to the unit for surgery, but died later that same day. They would be added as admissions and discharges, but the 11:59 p.m. census that night would still show 17 heads. The IPSDs, however, would be 19, which truly reflects the work done by the unit and the resources that were used.

HAPPY VALLEY HOSPITAL SURGICAL SERVICE: FEBRUARY 7, 2016

Adm/Disch	Census at Midnight	20
Admissions	+	5
Discharges	–	8
Patients at 11:59 p.m.	Total	17
A&D	+	2
IPSD	=	19

Of course, admissions and discharges are not the only way patients enter or leave a unit; patients are routinely transferred from one unit to another. Those will also need to be reflected in the unit census. While most hospitals use software to keep track of their census, an awareness of what that process looks like is important. Let us visualize what this would look like for a specific unit that includes transfers between units in the hospital and admissions, discharges, and deaths. Using a tabular format with the patient names, you can see where the figures for each of the numbers come from (Figure 4-3). Notice that the A&D same day (3) are for Shauna Blake (who was admitted and discharged), Louis Sterling (who was admitted and died), and Susan Summer (who was admitted and transferred out). Each of these patients was added to, and then

Happy Valley Memorial Hospital
April 15, 20XX
Surgical Unit

12 am Census ___24___

Admissions	Discharges
Sarah Cunningham	Andrew Washington
Shauna Blake	Selina Mark
Louis Sterling	Mason Morgan
Anthony Forester	Abbey Kruger
Susan Summer	Shauna Blake
	Siri Houston

Transfers In	Transfers Out
Nola Cumming	Susan Summer
Richard Foster	Dianna Hughes
Eva Fitzsimmons	Luther Nguyen
Freda Moore	

	Deaths
	Louis Sterling
	Rohan Pretz
	Joshua Brown

Beginning Census	24
Admissions	5
Transfers In	4
Subtotal	33
Discharges	6
Deaths	3
Transfers Out	3
11:59 p.m. Census	21
A&D Same Day	3
IPSD	24

Figure 4-3 The midnight census on the surgical unit of a hospital.

later subtracted from, the unit census. Without adding these three, the census calculation "loses" the services that the hospital provided to these patients.

Using a tabular format with the patient names, you can see where the figures for each of the numbers come from.

To provide another example, we could look at May 12th when there were 14 patients on the medical unit of Happy Valley Hospital. During the following 24 hours, there were three admissions, five patients discharged to home, one died, three individuals transferred to another unit, and two patients transferred in. One of the three admissions was the patient who died later that day. What is the 11:59 p.m. census on March 13?

To figure this out, we start with the beginning census of 14 and add in the new admissions (3) and the patients transferred in (2); $14 + 3 + 2 = 19$. From that subtotal, we subtract out the patients who left the unit: the five discharged to home, one death, and three patients transferred to another unit $(19 - (5 + 1 + 3) = 10)$. The census is then 10, but the inpatient service days are $10 + 1$ to include the one patient who was admitted and discharged (died) the same day. If the unit has two more patients that are admitted and discharged on the same day, then the IPSDs would be 13.

The inpatient census and IPSDs are **not** the same. The inpatient census is the actual number of patients in the hospital at census taking time, while IPSDs are a measure of the amount of work that the staff has done in treating patients during a census taking period. IPSDs are the census **plus** any patients who have been admitted and discharged on the same day.

Once the total number of IPSDs are calculated for a period of time, an average can be determined. The **average daily census** is the total number of IPSDs for a period divided by the days in the period. It gives an administrator a sense of how busy the hospital is for that particular period of time.

Average daily census The total number of IPSDs for a period divided by the days in the period.

Stat Tip

How many bed count days are there in a month? It depends on how many days that month has. The 31- and less-than-31-day months would be easy to remember if they simply alternated, but the pattern of month lengths is not that simple. They alternate until the fourth 31-day month, July, which is immediately followed by another 31-day month. Since the human hand has four fingers, one can, given an appropriate mind-set, perceive this pattern in a view of the knuckles of two fists, held together.

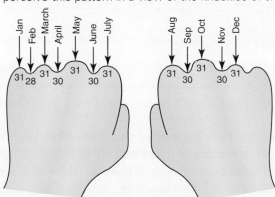

The raised knuckles can be seen as the 31-day months, the dips between them as the 30-day months and February, and the gap between the hands ignored. (Thus: left-hand-pinky-knuckle = January, dip = February, left-hand-ring-knuckle = March, dip = April, and so on to left-hand-index-knuckle = July; then continue with right-hand-index-knuckle = August, dip = September, etc.).

A simple poem can also help you remember the number of days in each month of the year:
Thirty days have September,
April, June, and November;
February has 28 alone,
All the rest have 31;
Except leap year, that's the time,
When February's days are 29.

Remember, when measuring the service that a hospital provides, the patients need to be admitted to qualify as part of the count. Outpatients, patients who arrive at the emergency department as DOA, and fetal deaths are not inpatients, so they are not included as an inpatient.

DOA Dead on arrival.

EXERCISE 4-2
Inpatient Census

1. The number of beds that are set up and staffed but not necessarily occupied are called the:

   a. Bed count
   b. Census
   c. Licensed beds
   d. Swing beds

2. Why is the bassinet count separate from the bed count?

3. The urology service has 14 patients at midnight on 2/7. Throughout the day of 2/8, there were four admissions and two discharges. What is the 2/8 census?

4. For the inpatient census on May 3, the hospital counts 149 adults and children and 12 newborns. That day, eight patients were admitted, two babies were born, two babies were discharged home, and one patient was transferred from another facility, but died the same day.

   a. Calculate the adult and child census for May 4.
   b. Calculate the newborn census for May 4.
   c. Calculate the IPSDs for May 4.

Occupancy

> **Occupancy** Is a ratio of the number of occupied beds to the number of available beds.

While the census tells us how many patients are in the facility, *occupancy* tells us how busy it is. Patient **occupancy** is a ratio of the number of occupied beds to the number of available beds. Usually expressed as a percentage, it is also called percentage of inpatient occupancy.

To calculate occupancy, we approach it the same way we would any other percentage, ratio, or rate—we are figuring out how much of a part we have of the whole. The part is the numerator, and the whole is the denominator. In this case, the part is how many patients we served (the IPSDs), and the whole is how many we *could* have treated (the bed count days). The formula for the percentage of occupancy looks like this:

> **IPSD** Inpatient service day.

Calculating Occupancy

$$\frac{\text{Total inpatient service days}}{\text{Total inpatient bed count days}} \times 100 = \% \text{ Occupancy}$$

Let us look at a simple example first. Say Happy Valley Hospital is a small facility licensed for 150 beds, and we want to know the occupancy for just one day, this past Monday. They staffed 100 beds on Monday (as they do most of the year), so this is the bed count, and since we are only looking at the occupancy for one day, we have a total of 100 bed count days. On that same day, we counted 75 patients in the census, and two patients who were admitted that same day died, for a total of 77 IPSDs. To set up the formula, see below:

$$\frac{\text{Total inpatient service days}}{\text{Total inpatient bed count days}} \times 100 = \% \text{ Occupancy} \quad \frac{77}{100} \times 100 = 77\%$$

The occupancy for Monday was 77%. Now, some things to note:

- Most of the time, the facility would be looking at occupancy rates over a longer period of time: a week, a month, a quarter, or a year. Occupancy rates for a single day fluctuate too much to be useful for planning services.
- The occupancy for adults and children is calculated separately from the bassinet occupancy rate. (It would have to be, since the bassinet count is separate from the bed count!)
- The percentage is usually expressed as a whole number.
- The calculation needs to take into account any changes in bed count to compare the number of beds that were actually occupied to those that were truly available for occupancy.

BRIEF CASE

COUNTING PATIENTS

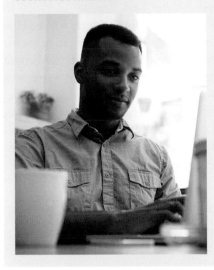

One of Michael's hospitals maintained 200 beds each day in the month of September, which has 30 days. The IPSDs for that period are 4250. He has two things he needs to figure out.

1. How many bed count days are there in September?

2. What is the occupancy rate for September at this hospital?

Some trickier calculations occur when there is a change in the bed count during the time period under observation. For example, imagine a hospital with 25 beds in a unit that never seemed to be at capacity. After much deliberation, the number of available beds was reduced to 15 in July, and remained at 15 for the rest of the year. The total IPSDs for that unit from January through June was 1800, and the total possible inpatient service days (the bed count) for those six months was $181 (31 + 28 + 31 + 30 + 31 + 30) \times 25 = 4525$. The occupancy rate for the first six months of the year is as follows:

$$\frac{1800}{25 \text{ (bed count)} \times 181 \text{ (days)}} \times 100 = 40\,\%$$

The total IPSDs for July through December was 1790, and the total possible IPSDs (i.e., the bed count days) for those second six months of the year was $(31 + 31 + 30 + 31 + 30 + 31) = 184 \times 15 = 2760$.

$$\frac{1790}{15 \text{ (bed count)} \times 184 \text{ (days)}} \times 100 = 65\,\%$$

After the reduction in beds in the unit, the occupancy rate rose to 65%. Once the facility reduced the number of beds, it saw a greater utilization of the resources it made available.

Now, how do we calculate the occupancy for this unit for the whole year, taking into account the change in bed count days? We add together the two separate calculations. The formula is as follows:

$$\frac{\text{Total inpatient service days } 1800 + 1790}{(25 \text{ (bed count)} \times 181 \text{ (days)}) + (15 \text{ (bed count)} \times 184 \text{ (days)})} \times 100 = 49\%$$

The total IPSDs was 1800 + 1790 = 3590, and the total possible IPSDs for the year was 4525 + 2760 = 7285. Dividing 3590 by 7285, you get 0.492793. Multiplying by 100 gives us 49% for the year.

There is no magic number for an ideal occupancy rate. The most recent statistics calculated through 2008 show an average occupancy rate among all hospitals nationwide of about 68%.[2] Acute care facilities would not want to plan for an occupancy that is too high because rates can and do fluctuate on a daily basis, and a facility would want to have beds available during an unexpectedly busy time. In fact, earlier in the chapter we mentioned that temporary and disaster beds are not included in the bed count. What would this mean in the case of a hurricane, for instance, when all the beds are full and a hospital might be forced to set up disaster beds in the waiting rooms and hallways? We would still count the patients treated in our IPSDs, but the bed count days would not change. This means it would be possible to have a figure in our numerator higher than the total in the denominator, i.e., an occupancy rate of greater than 100%!

Disasters and unusual circumstances aside, the industry trend these days is to limit inpatient care in an effort to lower costs. To that end, more patients are treated on an outpatient basis, and third party payers such as Medicare and insurance companies aim for shorter stays in the hospital. Table 4-2 shows the occupancy rates for US hospitals from 1975 to 2008.

MATH REVIEW

Remember that you always divide the actual numbers reported by the possible number. The multiplication by 100 will give you a percentage.

TABLE 4-2

OCCUPANCY RATES BY TYPE OF OWNERSHIP AND SIZE OF HOSPITAL: UNITED STATES, SELECTED YEARS, 1975–2008

TYPE OF OWNERSHIP AND HOSPITAL SIZE	1975	1980	1990	1995	2000	2007	2008
All hospitals	76.7	77.7	69.5	65.7	66.1	68.3	68.2
Federal	80.7	80.1	72.9	72.6	68.2	67.7	67.9
Non-federal	76.3	77.4	69.2	65.1	65.9	68.3	68.2
Community	75	75.6	66.8	62.8	63.9	66.6	66.4
Nonprofit	77.5	78.2	69.3	64.5	65.5	68.6	68.4
For profit	65.9	65.2	52.8	51.8	55.9	57.2	57.8
State/local government	70.4	71.1	65.3	63.7	63.2	66.5	66.1
6-24 beds	48	46.8	32.3	36.9	31.7	34.7	33.8
25-49 beds	56.7	52.8	41.3	42.6	41.3	46.2	46.7
50-99 beds	64.7	64.2	53.8	54.1	54.8	56.2	56.6
100-199 beds	71.2	71.4	61.5	58.8	60	61.8	61.9
200-299 beds	77.1	77.4	67.1	63.1	65	66.6	66.4
300-399 beds	79.7	79.7	70	64.8	65.7	69.6	69.4
400-499 beds	81.1	81.2	73.5	68.1	69.1	70.2	74.2
500 beds or more	80.9	82.1	77.3	71.4	72.2	75.8	74.9

Source: American Hospital Association (AHA) Annual Survey of Hospitals. Hospital Statistics, 1976, 1981, 1991–2010 editions. Chicago, IL. (Copyrights 1976, 1981, 1991–2010: Used with the permission of Health Forum LLC, an affiliate of the AHA.)

[2] http://www.cdc.gov/nchs/data/hus/2010/113.pdf.

EXERCISE 4-3
Occupancy

Use the table below to answer the following questions.

	MONTH	IPSDS	BED COUNT	OCCUPANCY %
1st Quarter	January	5500	200	
	February	5789	200	
	March	4700	200	
2nd Quarter	April	4920	200	
	May	4000	150	
	June	3780	150	
3rd Quarter	July	3991	150	
	August	3921	150	
	September	3568	150	
4th Quarter	October	3666	150	
	November	5000	200	
	December	5524	200	

1. There are 31 days in March. How many bed count days were there in that month? What was the occupancy rate?

2. There are 28 days in February for this year because it was not a leap year. What was the occupancy percentage that month?

3. There are 31 days in January, 28 days in February, and 31 days in March. What was this hospital's occupancy rate for the first quarter?

4. After the first month of the second quarter, this facility lowered the number of beds it set up and staffed. What was the total occupancy rate for the second quarter?

5. What was the occupancy rate for the whole year?

Length of Stay

Recognizing the number of patients that are in the hospital, while important, does not give a full picture of the hospital's service to the patients. **LOS** is a measure of how long the patient is using the facility's services. Again, most acute care facilities capture LOS digitally, but an understanding of where these figures come from is important.

LOS is measured from the day of admission to the day of discharge, and the days spent in the hospital are referred to as **discharge days**. (The LOS or the total LOS and the count of discharge days are exactly the same thing.) The actual day of discharge does not count as a full day spent in the hospital, so a patient admitted on Monday and discharged on Tuesday is said to have an LOS of one day, or one discharge day. It should be noted, however, that patients who are admitted and discharged the same day are considered to have a LOS of one.

IPSDs are counted while the patients are in the hospital. Discharge days are calculated after the patient is out of the hospital. Just like census, bed count, and occupancy statistics, LOS is also calculated separately for newborns because the newborns are accommodated in bassinets and the adults and children in beds.

Because the cost of hospitalizations is closely correlated to the length of stay, an average length of stay is a valuable statistic to calculate.

○ **Length of stay (LOS)** The duration of an inpatient visit, measured in whole days; the number of whole days between the inpatient's admission and discharge.

○ **Discharge days** The number of days a patient spends in the hospital.

○ **Average length of stay (ALOS)** The total number of discharge days for a group of patients being studied, then divided by the number of discharges in the group.

An **average length of stay (ALOS)** is the total number of discharge days for a group of patients being studied, then divided by the number of discharges in the group. Like all averages, the ALOS tells us how often something *usually* happens. An average length of stay for patients with a certain diagnosis, for example, is useful for projecting how long we might expect patients with the same diagnosis to be hospitalized. If the mean (average) LOS for all patients with appendicitis is 2.7 discharge days, then we can expect the patients at our hospital with an admitting diagnosis of appendicitis to stay about 2 or 3 days. As we will see shortly, the ALOS can also help us determine how often our hospital's beds free up for the next patient in a statistic called the *bed turnover rate*.

What if the ALOS at our hospital, or for the patients of a particular physician, varies from the mean? This might require further investigation. Let us say the ALOS for patients nationwide who underwent total or partial hip replacements is 4.1 discharge days. At our hospital, we ran a report by physician and procedure, and we calculate that over the past year, our hip replacement patients stayed an average of 4.5 days. The ALOS for most of our patients is 4 days, but Dr. Farley's patients tend to stay for 6.4 discharge days. There may be good reasons for this; perhaps Dr. Farley's patients are older, for example, and require longer recovery times. But such a variation from the mean would warrant review by the medical staff.

The Agency for Healthcare Quality Research and Quality (AHRQ) publishes the mean and median lengths of stay in their HCUPnet (http://hcupnet.ahrq.gov/). HCUPnet is a free, online query system based on data from the Healthcare Cost and Utilization Project (HCUP). It provides access to health statistics and information on hospital inpatient and emergency department utilization.

Leave of Absence Days

Sometimes, part of a patient's treatment includes a time period when he/she is not in the hospital. Long-term rehabilitation for some psychiatric, substance abuse, or other disorders that require extensive physical or occupational therapy may qualify for a short leave from the hospital. For example, a weekend "pass" may be given to allow the patient to use the skills they have acquired during their treatment to see how well they do at home. This time a patient spends outside the facility is called **leave of absence (LOA) days**. Because the days when the patient is out of the hospital are considered to be part of their treatment, they are included in their total LOS. LOA days do not count as IPSDs, however, because the patient is not present at census taking time.

○ **Leave of absence (LOA)** Days of time a patient spends outside the facility.

LOA days help differentiate the amount of time a patient underwent treatment from the amount of hospital resources that patient used. For example, say a patient is admitted on November 3 to a substance abuse rehabilitation facility. On November 24, he is granted a 48-hour pass to spend time with his family. He returns and is finally discharged on November 30. His total IPSDs are 25, while his total discharge days are 27.

TAKE AWAY ○ · · · · · · · ·

Leave of absence days are included in discharge days but are not included in IPSDs.

Bed Turnover Rate

Bed turnover rates give a sense of how often an individual bed changes its occupant during a given time period. Does the hospital have a few patients that stay for long periods of time? Or is the hospital experiencing a large number of patients that stay for shorter periods of time? Bed turnover measures how fast you get them in and get them out. This statistic has implications for virtually every function in the hospital. Certainly housekeeping needs to change the linens and prep rooms, but all of the admitting and discharging paperwork also figures in, in addition to the processing of records and bills. There are two standardized ways to calculate a bed turnover rate.

The *direct bed turnover rate* is the total number of discharges for a period divided by the average bed count for that same period. An example would be a hospital that has

600 discharges for the month of July with an average bed count of 150 beds. The direct bed turnover rate using this formula would be 600/150 = 4. This means that each bed changed occupants approximately four times during the month of July.

Another method of determining a turnover rate is called the *indirect bed turnover rate*. It has the occupancy rate (expressed as a decimal) multiplied by the number of days in the period in the numerator and the ALOS in the denominator. If a hospital had an 80% occupancy rate for the month of April and an ALOS for April of 3, the indirect bed turnover rate would be as follows:

$$\frac{0.80 \times 30}{3} = 8$$

In this example, this hospital had their beds change occupants eight times during the month of April. Notice that the direct rate uses IPSDs, while the indirect rate uses discharge days. They give slightly different numbers, because one measures turnover while the patients are in house, and the other measures retrospectively. Which formula you choose depends on whether you want to know what is happening concurrently, or if you want to look back historically.

EXERCISE 4-4
Length of Stay

Calculate the individual LOS for each of the following patients:

	ADMITTED	DISCHARGED	
1.	June 30	July 3	
2.	July 1	July 1	
3.	July 1	July 2	
4.	July 2	July 7	
5.	July 2	August 1	
6.	July 15	September 15	

7. Using the information above, how many discharge days were there in July?

8. What was the ALOS in July?

9. In June, a hospital counted 700 discharge days for its adults and children, and 125 discharges. It also had 51 newborn discharge days and 17 newborn discharges. What is the ALOS for adults and children? For newborns? What is the total ALOS?

10. A facility reports the following inpatient data for September:

Adults and Children	
Bed Count	100
Admissions	200
Discharges	220
IPSDs	1857
Discharge days	1837

a. What is the occupancy rate?
b. What is the direct bed turnover rate?
c. What is the indirect bed turnover rate to the thousandths place?

ALOS Average length of stay.

BRIEF CASE

COMPARING UTILIZATION

Michael needs to produce the statistics regarding average daily census (ADC), occupancy, and ALOS for each of the hospitals in the Diamonte system over the prior year. The system administrator has also asked for a table and graph that summarizes the data for occupancy. He checks the request for the time period required, opens the hospital system database, and sets up reports for each of the three hospitals in his system. What is the ALOS, ADC, and % Occupancy for both adults and children and newborns at each facility?

Happy Valley Hospital 2015	Adults and Children (A&C)	Newborns
Bed count	125	5
Admissions	14,477	874
Discharges	14,501	890
IPSDs	40,866	1537
Discharge days	42,555	1809

ALOS A&C	
ALOS NB	
ADC A&C	
ADC NB	
%Occupancy A&C	
%Occupancy NB	

St. Barnabas 2015	Adults and Children	Newborns
Bed count	90	5
Admissions	8912	998
Discharges	8960	1002
IPSDs	24,245	1234
Discharge days	29,452	1242

ALOS A&C	
ALOS NB	
ADC A&C	
ADC NB	
%Occ A&C	
%Occ NB	

Midtown General 2015	Adults and Children	Newborns
Bed count	250	25
Admissions	9593	902
Discharges	9600	905
IPSDs	36,011	4250
Discharge days	35,500	1501

ALOS A&C	
ALOS NB	
ADC A&C	
ADC NB	
%Occ A&C	
%Occ NB	

As he looks at the resulting tables, Michael has a sense of what he might find, and he decides to run a couple of quick graphs to attach to the reports. He notices that one of the hospitals seems to be reporting what could be a concern, so he quickly checks his calculations, builds a chart for occupancy, and sends off his findings to his boss. What does his bar chart look like?

1. How is outpatient care different from inpatient care? List some examples of both outpatient and inpatient settings.

2. Why is it important for each unit of a facility to take the census at the same time each day?

3. For the inpatient census on July 3, the hospital counts 90 adults and children and three newborns. That day, five patients were admitted, one baby was born, one patient was transferred to a nursing home, and one patient died in the emergency department. Calculate the adult and child and newborn census for July 4. Calculate the adult and child and newborn IPSDs.

4. Explain the difference between the census and the count of IPSDs.

5. One of the newborn units in the hospital reports its statistics for January as follows:

Bassinet count	8
Midnight census 1/1	5
Admissions	50
Discharged to home	49
Deaths	1
Total IPSDs	220

   a. How many bassinet count days are there in January?
   b. What is the newborn census at the end of January?
   c. What was the occupancy rate for this newborn unit in January?

6. What does the occupancy percentage tell us about the facility?

7. A facility reports the following inpatient data for October:

	Adults and Children	Newborns
Bed count	150	10
Admissions	455	30
Discharges	444	32
IPSDs	3601	125
Discharge days	3300	124

   Compute the following separately for adults and children and newborns:

	ADULTS AND CHILDREN	NEWBORNS
Bed count days		
Occupancy		
ALOS		
Direct bed turnover rate		
Indirect bed turnover rate to the thousandths place		

8. How do LOA days affect hospital statistics?

CLINICAL FACILITY DATA

CHAPTER OUTLINE

KEY TERMS

autopsy
complication
consultation
device days

fetal death
health care associated
    infections (HAI)
hospital-acquired condition (HAC)

miscarriage
morbidity
mortality
present on admission (POA)

LEARNING OBJECTIVES

At the end of the chapter, you should be able to do the following:

- Collect data on morbidity in health care settings and compute rates for infections and general complications.
- Explain and compute consultation rates.
- Define and calculate obstetric rates.
- Collect data on morbidity in health care settings and compute mortality rates for various patient populations.

- Define and calculate autopsy rates.
- Discuss trends in autopsy rates and calculate autopsy rates in health care.

The key products of the health care business are its treatments and outcomes. Much, if not most, of the data health care facilities collect on diagnoses, treatments, and outcomes can be used to assist in controlling costs and providing information regarding quality of care at a facility. Ideally, patients (and payers) would like to have the highest quality treatments with the best outcomes for the lowest cost. Clinical data can be used to help health care facilities, as well as consumers, to determine how a particular facility is scoring on a number of important measures to achieve those goals. This chapter will cover the most commonly used formulas to measure and summarize clinical data: *morbidity* statistics (dealing with diseases and disorders such as complications and infections), *mortality* statistics (deaths), a number of obstetrical statistics, consultation rates, and autopsies. The use of clinical data for cost issues is covered in Chapter 7, Departmental Data.

BRIEF CASE

PREPARING VITAL STATS

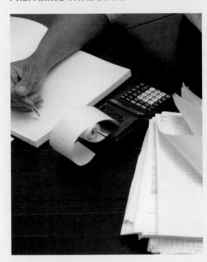

Opening his email, Michael finds the first order of business for the day: a request from the Surgical Department for a Morbidity and Mortality (M&M) conference later in the week. The request includes a comparison of a variety of M&M measures regarding the outcomes of the hospital's bariatric surgeries. Michael eyeballs his bookshelf to look for his old stat book, stretches, and reaches for a pad of paper to write down the exact rates required.

● **M&M** Morbidity and Mortality.

This chapter will cover the specific rates used to measure clinical data in a facility. All of the rates we discuss in this chapter use the basic rate formula you reviewed in Chapter 2. If you remember, every time we are looking at the rate of an occurrence, we are talking about the number of times a thing occurred out of (divided by) the number times it *could have* occurred. Thinking back to numerators and denominators, our rates always compare what actually happened, compared to what could have happened.

✎ Calculating a Basic Rate

$$\frac{\text{Number of times something occurred in a time period}}{\text{Number of times it could have occurred in the same time period}} \times 100 = \text{rate}$$

We then standardize our rates for comparison by multiplying them by a constant, usually 100, to express the result as a percent. So to get started on the rates in this chapter, let us say someone has 10 fish in a fish tank and discovers that 2 of them died last week. What is the *mortality rate* (the death rate) for the aquarium last week?

$$\frac{\text{2 fish died last week}}{\text{10 fish could have died last week}} \times 100 = 20\% \text{ fish mortality rate}$$

● MATH REVIEW

If 2 of the fish continue to die each week, then the mortality rate will climb each week (2/8 or 25%, 2/6 or 33%, 2/4, or 50%, and 2/2, 100%). Notice that the denominator is of the remaining fish each week. After week 5, there are no fish left that could possibly die, so the formula becomes irrelevant. The tank will be empty in just a few weeks.

Aside from the fact that the fish mortality rate is kind of high, did you notice the time periods in the numerator and denominator? We calculated the mortality rate using data from *within the same time frame*. Those time periods are important because a lot of the work that a data analyst does is in comparisons, which may be required in weekly, monthly, quarterly, or annual formats. Hopefully, those comparisons will show an improvement in a rate.

MORBIDITY RATES

Measuring Complications

In the Brief Case at the start of this chapter, Michael was getting ready for an M&M conference. These conferences, held routinely at many medical centers, tend to focus on a small number of patients whose treatments resulted in a negative outcome or who were involved in a suspected medical error, or whose case provided an opportunity to learn. The presentations may focus on the types of diseases and disorders present upon the patients' admissions and the treatments provided. Or, more likely, they address the diseases or disorders that patients developed while staying at the hospital—diseases or disorders that may have been the result of their treatment. **Hospital-acquired conditions (HACs)** are those conditions that occur *after* a patient has been admitted to the hospital. For example, an HAC might be a consequence of a particular device that is used in surgery, and health care providers are interested in tracking how often these devices cause problems. Health care providers track HAC and other morbidity rates to improve treatment and outcome quality, and to lower costs.

Payers are interested in morbidity rates as well. The Centers for Medicare and Medicaid (CMS), along with other third-party payers (health insurers), view HACs as preventable conditions. Accordingly, these payers do not want to compensate health care providers for the treatment of a disease or disorder that would not have occurred if the health care facility used appropriate care. One example is a condition called pressure ulcers, or bed sores. A pressure ulcer is a type of skin damage that occurs mostly among patients who have limited mobility, when the soft tissue of the body is compressed between the bones and an external surface (e.g., a bed) for an extended period of time. Since the more severe grades of pressure ulcers can be prevented by helping the patient turn every two hours (Fig. 5-1), third-party payers will not compensate the facility for the costs to treat this HAC.

After the passing of the Deficit Reduction Act of 2005, CMS required reporting of HAC and **present on admission (POA)** indicators for all inpatient discharges. POA indicators are conditions a patient has upon admission; they are coded as the principal

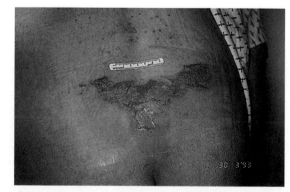

Figure 5-1 Pressure ulcers, a common hospital-acquired condition (HAC), can be prevented by regular turning of the patient.

or secondary diagnosis, and a record of POAs is required for all Medicare inpatient admissions to an inpatient hospital. This requirement aims to determine whether a patient entered the health care facility with a disease or disorder, or whether the patient developed the condition while in the facility. If a patient is discharged with a *new* diagnosis that is an HAC, the hospital *will not be reimbursed* for the treatment of that condition.

This means that not only does a hospital have an interest in providing quality care because it is the right thing to do for the patient, but because it will lose money if it does not. Facilities monitor the rates of HACs and complications carefully. According to the MS-DRG system of reimbursement, a **complication** is any adverse event that happens to a patient after admission to the hospital that causes an increase in the length of stay by at least one day, in 75% of the patients. Examples of complications could be a sponge left in a patient after surgery, incorrectly administering a medication that causes harm, a fall out of bed, an infection after surgery, or a serious bed sore, as discussed above. Box 5-1 lists the HAC categories for which CMS will not pay as of fiscal year (FY) 2015.

> **Complication** An adverse event that happens to a patient after admission to the hospital that causes an increase in the length of stay by at least one day, in 75% of the patients.

BOX 5-1   CMS NON-REIMBURSABLE HAC CATEGORIES FOR FISCAL YEAR (FY) 2015

- Foreign object retained after surgery air embolism
- Blood incompatibility
- Pressure ulcer stages III & IV
- Falls and trauma:
  - Fracture
  - Dislocation
  - Intracranial injury
  - Crushing injury
  - Burn
  - Other injuries
- Catheter-associated urinary tract infection (UTI)
- Manifestations of poor glycemic control:
  - Diabetic ketoacidosis
  - Non-ketotic hyperosmolar coma
  - Hypoglycemic coma
  - Secondary diabetes with ketoacidosis
  - Secondary diabetes with hyperosmolarity
- SSIs, mediastinitis, following coronary artery bypass graft (CABG)
- SSIs following certain orthopedic procedures:
  - Spine
  - Neck
  - Shoulder
  - Elbow
- SSIs following bariatric surgery for obesity:
  - Laparoscopic gastric bypass
  - Gastroenterostomy
  - Laparoscopic gastric restrictive surgery
- SSIs following cardiac implantable
- Electronic device (CIED)
- Deep vein thrombosis and pulmonary embolism following certain orthopedic procedures:
  - Total knee replacement
  - Hip replacement
- Iatrogenic pneumothorax with venous catheterization

Stat Tip

Not every infection or medication error will be classified as a complication or an HAC. Care must be taken to categorize events as complications. Each should be under the purview of a physician.

● MATH REVIEW

Like all rate calculations, this rate is the number of times something occurred, out of (divided by) the number times it *could have* occurred. The numerator is the number of patients with the morbidity under study, and the denominator is the number of discharges for the same time period.

TAKE AWAY ●··········

CMS and other third-party payers will not reimburse providers for certain types of HACs.

To measure a morbidity (an HAC or complication) rate, you divide the number of complications by the number of discharges:

✏ Measuring Morbidity

$$\frac{\text{Total number of complications in a time period}}{\text{Total number of discharges (including deaths) in a time period}} \times 100$$

Notice here, that we are using discharges in the denominator. Some hospitals use admissions data instead. How do you know when to use admissions versus when to use discharges? Admissions in the denominator would be for concurrent stats, while discharged patients give retrospective statistics. The advantage of concurrent stats is that one can act on the data and improve conditions for current patients; however "real-time" concurrent statistics are not often available and are more difficult to use for benchmarking purposes.

The diagnoses associated with all these complications and more are monitored statistically by CMS, so each complication is usually calculated in more specific detail, rather than as HACs as a whole. To calculate the rate for each of the cases listed in Box 5-1, simply substitute the condition (burn, fracture, retained foreign object) in the numerator and compare it to the possibility for that condition to occur to either admission or discharges in the denominator.

How often do HACs happen? Both providers and payers expect these cases to be quite rare. These numbers are usually smaller than the infection rates discussed below and are often expressed as occurrences per 1000 patients instead of as percentages.

BRIEF CASE

FINDING THE COMPLICATION RATE

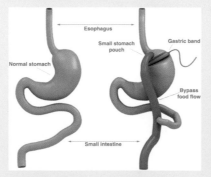

Gastric bypass surgery methods.

Physicians need to have metrics on complications, so that the best possible techniques and measures can be used to prevent them in the future. Data analytics can provide the valuable feedback required. Michael's review of the literature regarding gastric bypass complications yielded the study below: a summary of complications of gastric bypass surgery after a 14-year period. 312 surgeries were performed, and a complete follow-up was obtained for 178 patients. Notice that the complications are varied in nature: infections (gastritis, cholecystitis), nutritional (vitamin B_{12} deficiency, dehydration), mental health (depression), and several are related to complications of the surgery itself (staple line failure, incisional hernia). Calculate the complication rate for each disorder experienced by patients during the 14-year follow-up.

Continued

BRIEF CASE—cont'd

GASTRIC BYPASS SURGERY COMPLICATION: 14-YEAR FOLLOW-UP

COMPLICATION	CASES	RESULT	RATE
Vitamin B$_{12}$ deficiency	52		
Incisional hernia	51		
Depression	41		
Staple line failure	39		
Gastritis	24		
Cholecystitis	19		
Dehydration	12		
Dilated pouch	4		

Measuring Health Care Associated Infections (HAIs)

In 2011, the CDC reported that "on any given day, about one in 25 hospital patients has at least one healthcare-association infection" and that "75,000 hospital patients with HAIs (hospital-acquired infections) died during their hospitalizations."[1]

In the history of medicine, before physicians understood the microorganisms that cause disease, there was a time when patients preferred to stay out of hospitals if they could. The combination of poor hygiene by hospital staff and the collection of so many sick patients in one place meant that you were likely to leave the hospital sicker than you arrived—provided you were able to leave at all.

Today, we understand the viruses, fungi, and bacteria that cause infection, but the danger of contracting an infectious disease while hospitalized remains, and it is a primary concern for every facility. Hospital staffs take great care to ensure a clean environment, which includes proper hand-washing and hygiene, various levels of isolation for patients with highly-communicable diseases, and of course, the sterilization of instruments.

HAIs, also called *nosocomial* infections, are one of the many HACs discussed previously, but they have their own sets of formulas. A division of the CDC, the National Healthcare Safety Network (NHSN), tracks HAIs in both outpatient and inpatient settings and makes the information available to patients and the facilities themselves. HAIs may be categorized as surgical site infections (SSIs), central line-associated bloodstream infections (CLABSIs) (Fig. 5-2), or have the name of a specific pathogen (MRSA, VRSA, or *C. diff*).

The reasons for such tracking and precautions are evident. If a patient is admitted to the hospital for a broken hip and contracts pneumonia during her stay, she will likely take a longer time to recover, stay in the hospital longer, and her conditions will cost more to treat. As discussed above, Medicare and other insurers will decline to pay for the treatment of certain HAIs, such as a urinary tract infection (UTI) following catheterization. Besides the threat to the individual patient, facilities worry about the spread of disease to other patients as well. Many patients in the hospital are immunocompromised due to advanced age, AIDS, or other diseases that affect the immune system, and certain treatments like chemotherapy.

So how does a hospital measure HAI rates? If the rates are very tiny (less than 1%), they may be multiplied by a larger constant to yield a rate per 1000. For example, an overall infection rate last week at a facility might be four out of 100 or 4%. But if the

Health care associated infections (HAIs) Infections developed during the course of treatment.

HAC Hospital-acquired condition.

CDC Centers for Disease Control and Prevention.

NHSN National Healthcare Safety Network.

SSI Surgical site infection.

CLABSI Central line-associated bloodstream infection.

UTI Urinary tract infection.

TAKE AWAY •·········

HAIs increase health care delivery costs.

[1] http://www.cdc.gov/hai/surveillance/.

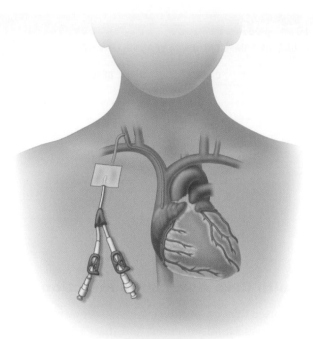

Figure 5-2 A central line catheter is a long, thin tube inserted to deliver medication, fluids, or blood over a longer period of time than an IV would normally be used. Although there are different kinds, they all share the possibility of an associated bloodstream infection: hence the need to measure the number of CLABSIs in an institution.

hospital was interested in examining their rate of SSIs alone, it might only be two in 1000 cases (2/1000 or what would have been 0.2%).

> ## Stat Tip
> Since these rates are used to measure the change of the size of the infection rate (hopefully in a negative direction), you must be sure to continue to use the formulas already in use by the hospital. If they measure in patients per 1000 instead of as a percent—or measure in inpatient service days instead of by the patient—make sure you do the same. Otherwise, your reports may yield (or miss) some alarming information.

How can we tell if the patient acquired an infection in the hospital, as opposed to having the infection before she was admitted? While a patient may not have a visibly present infection on admission, it may be incubating. The CDC defines HAIs as those that occur more than 48 to 72 hours after admission, and within 10 days after discharge. If a patient is admitted on Monday and shows symptoms of pneumonia on Tuesday, they probably had pneumonia prior to admission, and it probably should not be counted "against" the hospital. If the infection manifests on Thursday, on the other hand, it is counted in the hospital's HAI rates. This is a case where you will need to check your hospital's past practice or written guidelines to find out how they want these infections counted.

 Calculating an HAI Rate

$$\frac{\text{Total number of infections after 48 (or 72 hours) of hospitalization for a period}}{\text{Total number of discharges (including deaths) for a period}} \times 100$$

Unfortunately, some patients may develop more than one infection, so your numerator could measure either infections, or numbers of infected patients. State departments of health provide guidelines instructing practitioners how and when to count multiple infections in one patient. Remember that these are infections that the patient did not have (or were not identified) on admission.

If your health care facility wants to measure the number of HAIs present during a month of discharged patients, the formula would be:

 Calculating an Infection Rate

$$\frac{\text{Total number of infections in a given month}}{\text{Total number of patients discharged for the same month}} \times 100$$

Be careful to compare the patient population to the number of infections that could have happened in that population. For example, if you wanted to look at the number of infections present in your population of Medicare patients, be sure to compare infections in Medicare patients to only your Medicare patient population, not the patient population as a whole. The rate would be much smaller if you mistakenly use a denominator that is inappropriate for your numerator.

Surgical Site Infections (SSIs)

The most common type of hospital infection is an SSI. In 2010, CDC reported 31% of all hospital-acquired infections were SSIs, so hospitals monitor the rates of infection following surgical procedures closely. Because dirty wounds become infected more readily than clean ones, a classification of wounds, adapted from the American College of Surgeons, is used to determine if the incision for the procedure is clean or contaminated (Table 5-1). The formula used to calculate SSIs among clean surgical cases is as follows:

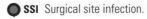 **SSI** Surgical site infection.

 Calculating a Postoperative Infection Rate

$$\frac{\text{Total number of postoperative infections}}{\text{Total number of clean surgical procedures}} \times 100$$

Stat Tip

As always, make sure that you are comparing the numerator time unit (per week, per month, per year) to the same time unit in the denominator. The best way to decide the constant is to take your lead from previously reported rates. They can serve as your guide as to the previous magnitude of the result and the constant that was used (multiplying by 100 for a percent or by 1000 to make your dividend greater than one.)

Infections Caused by Use of Devices

Because infections may be related to the use of devices that are used to treat a specific disease (ventilators, for example, as seen in Fig. 5-3), additional rates are often calculated to measure infections that accompany their use. Pneumonia, for instance, is a commonly-occurring HAI, and it is particularly dangerous because hospital-acquired pneumonia (HAP) can be more resistant to antibiotics than other types. A subset of HAP is ventilator-associated pneumonia (VAP), which can develop when infectious

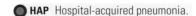 **HAP** Hospital-acquired pneumonia.

VAP Ventilator-acquired pneumonia.

TABLE 5-1

SURGICAL WOUND CLASSIFICATION

CLASS	CLASSIFICATION	DESCRIPTION
Class I	Clean	An uninfected operative wound in which no inflammation is encountered, and the respiratory, alimentary, genital, or uninfected urinary tract is not entered. In addition, clean wounds are primarily closed and, if necessary, drained with closed drainage. Operative incisional wounds that follow non-penetrating (blunt) trauma should be included in this category if they meet the criteria.
Class II	Clean-contaminated	An operative wound in which the respiratory, alimentary, genital, or urinary tracts are entered under controlled conditions and without unusual contamination. Specifically, operations involving the biliary tract, appendix, vagina, and oropharynx are included in this category, provided no evidence of infection or major break in technique is encountered.
Class III	Contaminated	Open, fresh, accidental wounds. In addition, operations with major breaks in sterile technique (e.g., open cardiac massage) or gross spillage from the gastrointestinal tract, and incisions in which acute, non-purulent inflammation is encountered are included in this category.
Class IV	Dirty-infected	Old traumatic wounds with retained devitalized tissue and those that involve existing clinical infection or perforated viscera. This definition suggests that the organisms causing postoperative infection were present in the operative field before the operation.

From Garner, JS. CDC guideline for prevention of surgical wound infections, 1985. Supercedes guideline for prevention of surgical wound infections published in 1982. (Originally published in 1985). Revised. Infect Control 1986; 7(3):193–200.

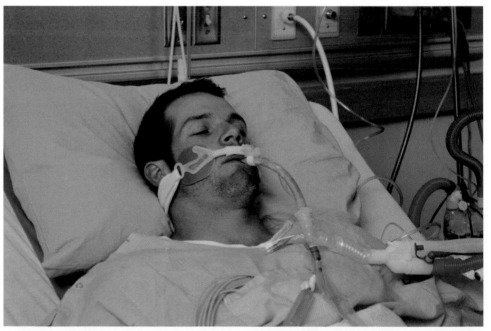

Figure 5-3 The use of a ventilator can lead to ventilator-associated pneumonia (VAP), which can develop when infectious agents in the environment reach the lower airways through the ventilator tube.

agents in the environment reach the lower airways through the ventilator tube. The formula to calculate the VAP rate is:

 Calculating VAP in Discharged Patients

$$\frac{\text{Patients with VAP for a time period}}{\text{Discharged patients who were on a mechanical ventilator for a time period}} \times 100$$

This formula lets you know how many of your patients on a ventilator are developing pneumonia while being treated in your facility.

Device Use Rates

Statistics connecting HAIs to devices may be more meaningful in the context of how often the device was used in your patient population. To measure ventilator usage, we divide the number of patients who used a ventilator by the total number of patients:

 Calculating Ventilator Usage

$$\frac{\text{Patients on mechanical ventilators for a time period}}{\text{Patients discharged for a time period}} \times 100$$

In addition to ventilators, SSIs may involve devices. Although the infections are usually at the surface of the skin, they may also be associated with bariatric surgery for obesity, or more recently, following the placement of a cardiac implantable electronic device (CIED). Other devices that can cause infections include central line catheters and urinary catheters.

Often, the amount of time a patient uses a device correlates to the incidence of infection. Data analysts use the concept of **device days**, a measure of the opportunity for an infection to take place with a greater exposure to the use of the device. If, for example, we wanted to know ventilator days in a facility, we would count the number of patients using a ventilator for a particular number of days. Rates calculated with device days take into account the exposure of the patients over time, as opposed to just the presence or absence of an infection in the patient population. An example of this rate formula is:

 Calculating Infection Rate Compared to Days on Ventilator

$$\frac{\text{Patients with VAP for a time period}}{\text{Ventilator days for a time period}} \times 100$$

EXERCISE 5-1

Morbidity Rates

1. When calculating retrospective rates, the number of _____ is in the denominator.

2. Of 12,282 patients, 552 had one or more health care associated infections. Of 604 such infections, the most common type was pneumonia, accounting for 22.18%. How many pneumonia infections were there?

TAKE AWAY

Infections following surgeries and the use of medical devices are tracked in health care to both improve the quality of treatment and lower health care delivery costs.

HAI Health care associated infection.

Device days The number of patients using a device for a particular number of days.

EXERCISE 5-1
Morbidity Rates—cont'd

3. Out of 89 hip surgeries and 101 knee surgeries performed this year, 19 patients experienced complications. What is the complication rate? Round to the nearest whole number.

Use the following year-end data to calculate the requested statistics. Round to the nearest whole number.

    513 patients with HAIs
    97 patients with VAP
    6824 discharges
    431 patients on ventilators
    3017 ventilator days

4. Calculate the percentage of patients with VAP using ventilator days.

5. Calculate the percentage of patients with HAIs.

6. Calculate the percentage of patients on ventilators that develop VAP.

CONSULTATION RATE

Consultation The formal request by a physician for the professional opinion or services of another heath care professional, usually another physician, in caring for a patient.

Sometimes a physician must consult with another physician regarding the care of a patient. If the attending physician in charge of a patient's care plan needs more expertise or help treating a certain disorder or condition, he or she can request a **consultation** with another doctor. For example, if a patient who is admitted for a heart condition also has diabetes, the attending physician may make a formal request for the patient to be evaluated by an endocrinologist. The endocrinologist then evaluates the patient and responds to the request with specific diagnostic or therapeutic options and recommendations. Such reports become part of the medical record, and consultation rates are tracked because they represent additional care (and cost) in the treatment of a particular patient/diagnosis.

One patient can be seen by more than one consulting physician. Our patient with a heart condition and diabetes may very well have problems with his feet and require examination by a podiatrist, or may have stomach pains and need to be seen by a gastroenterologist. Because of this, there are two ways to calculate consultation rates: one shows the number of patients who received one or more consultations; the other shows the number of consultations that were provided. Each formula is listed below.

 Calculating Consultation Rates Using Total Number of Patients Seen

$$\frac{\text{Total number of patients seen by a consultant}}{\text{Total number of discharges (including deaths)}} \times 100$$

 Calculating Consultation Rates Using Total Number of Consultations

$$\frac{\text{Total number of consultations (reports) provided}}{\text{Total number of discharges (including deaths)}} \times 100$$

EXERCISE 5-2

Consultation Rates

Use the following year-end data to calculate the requested statistics. Provide answers rounded to the nearest whole number.

815 patients seen by consultants

9743 discharges

2409 consultations

1. Calculate the consultation rate of patients seen.
2. Calculate the rate of consultations provided.

OBSTETRIC RATES

Almost four million babies were born in hospitals in 2012—the number one diagnosis for the year! (Pneumonia trailed a distant second with approximately one million cases.) Birth rates are of interest to hospitals and to state and federal authorities. Hospitals need to keep track of birth rates so that they can have adequate staff and facilities to handle the workload. The government is interested in obstetric rates to monitor population growth and provide for the care of these new citizens. The formulas used for each of these obstetric rates, however, is different.

Hospitals "admit" newborns through the act of their birth at their facilities, or put another way, babies admit themselves to the hospital by the act of being born. A hospital's birth rate is calculated from these newborn admissions to a hospital.

The American Academy of Pediatrics (AAP) defines a birth as the "complete expulsion or extraction from the mother of a product of human conception, irrespective of the duration of pregnancy, which, after such expulsion or extraction, breathes or shows any other evidence of life, such as beating of the heart, pulsation of the umbilical cord, or definite movement of voluntary muscles, regardless of whether the umbilical cord has been cut or the placenta is attached. Heartbeats are to be distinguished from transient cardiac contractions; respirations are to be distinguished from fleeting respiratory efforts or gasps." While that seems like a long definition, it provides a definition that divides a live born from a fetal death. Statistics are kept separately for each of these categories that are not only national, but are also collected by the World Health Organization to compare international trends.

AAP defines a **fetal death** as one in which death occurs "before the complete expulsion or extraction from the mother of a product of human conception, irrespective of the duration of pregnancy, that is not an induced termination of pregnancy. The death is indicated by the fact that, after such expulsion or extraction, the fetus does not breathe or show any other evidence of life such as beating of the heart, pulsation of the umbilical cord, or definite movement of voluntary muscles. Heartbeats are to be distinguished from transient cardiac contractions; respirations are to be distinguished from fleeting respiratory efforts or gasps."

For statistical purposes, fetal deaths are further subdivided as "early" (20 to 27 weeks' gestation) or "late" (≥28 weeks' gestation).* The term "stillbirth" is also used to describe fetal deaths at 20 weeks' gestation or more. According to the AAP, fetuses that die in utero before 20 weeks' gestation are not considered fetal deaths; they are categorized specifically as **miscarriages**. Early fetal deaths are seldom reported, although a 2012 study in the National Vital Statistics Reports publication demonstrates that the majority of fetal deaths occur before 20 weeks.

AAP American Academy of Pediatrics.

Fetal death The un-induced death of a fetus before extraction from the mother.

Miscarriage A fetal death before 20 weeks' gestation.

*The World Health Organization (WHO) breaks fetal deaths into three periods; they define early as <20 weeks, intermediate as 20-27 weeks, and 28+ weeks as late.

While AAP has a standardized set of definitions for reporting of fetal deaths, various states use a variety of definitions for their reporting. Some states consider only the age of the fetus, while others only take the weight of the fetus into consideration. Still others combine age with a certain weight. For example:

- In Pennsylvania, the fetus must be older than 16 weeks to be considered a fetal death. In Puerto Rico, it must be older than 5 months.
- In Delaware, Kansas, and Montana, the fetus must be over 350 grams. In New Mexico, South Dakota, and Tennessee, it must be over 500 grams to be classified as a fetal death.
- In Arizona, Idaho, Kentucky, Louisiana, Massachusetts, Mississippi, Missouri, New Hampshire, South Carolina, Wisconsin, and Guam, the fetus must be older than 20 weeks and over 350 grams in weight. In the District of Columbia, it must be older than 20 weeks and over 500 grams.

Statistics on induced abortions are classified and calculated separately from other types of fetal death. AAP defines an induced abortion as the "purposeful interruption of an intrauterine pregnancy with the intention other than to produce a live-born infant and which does not result in a live birth." These are reported separately from the spontaneous abortions (un-induced), stillbirths, and miscarriages.

 Calculating the Fetal Death Rate

$$\frac{\text{Total number of fetal deaths for a period}}{\text{Total number of births} + \text{fetal deaths for this period}} \times 100$$

The denominator in the rate calculation includes all births in addition to all fetal deaths of the age under consideration.

 CS Cesarean section.

Cesarean Section (CS) Rates

The method of delivery is generally divided into vaginal or CS births. In the past, CSs were performed only in extreme cases to save the life of the mother or the baby. CSs became more commonplace over time, and were often requested on the part of the mother or the physician. Today, hospitals monitor their CS rates and review for medical necessity. The American College of Obstetricians and Gynecologists has expressed concern that an unnecessary first CS may lead to later complications with repeat procedures. As of 2012, the CDC reported that 32.8% of all deliveries were by CS, a 60% increase since the mid-1990s.

 Calculating CS Rates

$$\frac{\text{Total number of Ceserean sections for a period}}{\text{Total number of deliveries (live or dead) for this period}} \times 100$$

Another rate that is often calculated is the vaginal birth after Cesarean section (VBAC) rate. Although the earlier method of performing a CS resulted in an increased risk for subsequent vaginal births, the newer transverse incision allows for vaginal births after a CS. The rate for this is calculated as follows:

Calculating VBAC Rates

TAKE AWAY

CS rates are tracked and reviewed for medical necessity.

$$\frac{\begin{array}{c}\text{Total number vaginal deliveries among}\\ \text{women who had prior Cesarean sections}\end{array}}{\begin{array}{c}\text{Total number of Cesarean section births among}\\ \text{women who had prior Cesarean sections}\end{array}} \times 100$$

Maternal Mortality Rate (MMR)

A mortality is a death. The MMR is also referred to as the pregnancy-related mortality rate or obstetric mortality rate. The CDC uses the term "pregnancy-related death rate," and this rate includes deaths that are both direct (specifically caused by pregnancy or delivery, such as a uterine hemorrhage during delivery) or indirect (a condition that is exacerbated by the pregnancy such as hypertension, diabetes, or chronic heart disease). It does not include deaths that are not related to the pregnancy, such as a car accident—those types or deaths would be termed nonmaternal deaths.

In the United States, like most of the developed world, the number of women who died during childbirth dropped sharply during the last century due to medical advances, including aseptic techniques and prenatal care. Calculating maternal death rates in a hospital today should yield a percentage that is extremely low. As a matter of fact, the rate is usually accompanied by one of the largest constants: 100,000. As of 2012, the CIA reported the United States with a rate of 21 maternal deaths per 100,000, compared to a low of two per 100,000 in Estonia and 1100 per 100,000 in Chad.

 Calculating Maternal Mortality Rates

The denominator in the rate calculation should include only discharges of women from the obstetrical or maternity wards. It should be noted that the World Health Organization uses a formula that compares maternal deaths to live births instead of obstetrical discharges. Again, check with your hospital as to the particular rate that they have been using.

$$\frac{\text{Total number of maternal deaths for a period}}{\text{Total number of discharges from the OB wards (including deaths) for this period}} \times 100$$

> **TAKE AWAY** ●·········
>
> Because maternal mortalities are so rare, a large constant (100,000) is often used to express meaningful results.

Newborn Mortality Rate

The newborn mortality rate measures the total number of deaths of babies from birth up to the first year of life.

 Calculating Newborn Mortality Rates

$$\frac{\text{Total number of newborn deaths for a period}}{\text{Total number of newborn discharges (including deaths) for this period}} \times 100$$

Neonatal Mortality Rate

The neonatal mortality rate compares the number of deaths of newborns under the age of 28 days compared to the number of newborn discharges. An early, more targeted neonatal mortality rate measures deaths in the first seven days of life. A late neonatal mortality rate measures deaths from seven to 28 days of life.

 Calculating Neonatal Mortality Rates

$$\frac{\text{Total number of neonatal deaths for a period}}{\text{Total number of neonatal discharges (including deaths) for this period}} \times 100$$

> ## Stat Tip ··
>
> The term newborn is sometimes used interchangeably with the term neonatal, but this is incorrect; the two words mean different things. When calculating, be sure which of the newborn rates is required.

EXERCISE 5-3

Obstetric Rates

Use the following year-end data to calculate the requested statistics. Provide your answers in whole numbers.

    167 deliveries
    182 live births
    42 CSs
    3 VBACs

1. Given 7 early and 4 late fetal deaths and 856 live births, what is the fetal death rate rounded to one decimal place?

2. Calculate the CS rate.

3. Calculate the VBAC rate.
   Use the following year-end data to calculate the requested statistics. Round your answers to two decimal places.
   5 newborn deaths
   3 neonatal deaths
   317 newborn discharges
   1 pregnancy-related death
   479 obstetrical discharges

4. Calculate the newborn mortality rate.

5. Calculate the neonatal mortality rate.

MORTALITY RATES

● **Mortality** Death.

Mortality rates measure the numbers and percentages of deaths in a hospital for a specific time period. The rate can be hospital-wide, or it can be calculated for specific diagnoses, procedures, services, or individual physicians. A 2010 study showed that 29% of all deaths occurred in hospitals, but did not account for the severity of admitting diagnoses or the ages of the patients. The graph in Figure 5-4 from the CDC shows the decrease in hospital deaths over the last decade, with fewer patients dying in a hospital setting. Whether this means that the patients are dying in nursing facilities or at home is another topic to be studied, but the deaths are significantly fewer.

Measuring Gross and Net Mortality Rates

Hospitals have two ways of calculating their mortality rates: gross and net mortality rates. The *gross mortality rate* is the number of inpatient deaths divided by the number of discharges. Admissions to the hospital do not include patients who were dead on arrival (DOA) or patients who died in an outpatient or emergency department setting.

● **DOA** Dead on arrival.

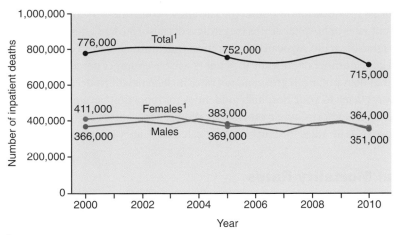

¹Significant decrease from 2000 to 2010.
Note: Statistical significance was measured using a weighted least-squares regression method, including data from all years, to measure linear trends over time.
Source: CDC/NCHS, National Hospital Discharge Survey, 2000-2010

Figure 5-4 Inpatient hospital deaths: United States, 2000–2010.

Because this rate could be used to reflect on the quality of care at a hospital (would you want to be admitted to a hospital with a high mortality rate?), it does not make sense to hold patients who were DOA, or deaths of outpatients or ED patients against the inpatient hospital results. The rate includes all deaths, meaning adults and children, along with newborns, unless stated otherwise.

 ED Emergency department.

The *net mortality rate* also includes the inpatient deaths divided by the discharges, but it subtracts the number of inpatient deaths that occurred under 48 hours. Remember that the same exclusions and inclusions for the gross mortality rate apply here also.

Calculating Gross Mortality Rates

$$\frac{\text{Total number of inpatient deaths}}{\text{Total number of discharges (including deaths)}} \times 100$$

Calculating Net Mortality Rates

$$\frac{\text{Total number of inpatient deaths (including newborns)} - \text{deaths } <48 \text{ hours after admission}}{\text{Total number of discharges (including newborns)} - \text{deaths } <48 \text{ hours after admission}} \times 100$$

Stat Tip ·································

You can think about *gross* and *net* rates the same way we think of gross earnings and net earnings. Gross income refers to the total amount before any reductions, while net income is the amount you take home. Net income does not show the total amount you earned, but it is a more realistic calculation of the amount of money you have to spend. In the same way, the net mortality rate is a more realistic calculation of the patients who died under the care of the facility.

The reason for the net rate is to allow for a comparison of deaths to discharges where the time period allows for the hospital to perform treatment. Although the standard formula uses 48 hours, Hospital Compare, Medicare's quality database, uses 30 days instead of

48 hours for its statistics cut off point. The site allows consumers to compare hospitals that have different rates of hospital deaths (regardless of cause) 30 days after admission for three specific diagnoses: acute myocardial infarction, pneumonia, and heart failure. Hospitals that treat a large number of critically ill patients will have a larger percentage of deaths than a hospital that does not. Both gross and net rates include newborn deaths, unless otherwise stated. Always defer to your hospital's guidelines for reporting because some may require the inclusion of newborns, while others may require separate statistics for adults/children and newborns. Death rates for outpatients, if calculated, are performed separately.

Surgical Mortality Rates

Gross and net death rates gives an overview, but they are not especially helpful as to where or under what circumstances the deaths are occurring in the hospital setting. Two of the most common specialty death rates are the postoperative (postop) death rate and the anesthesia death rate.

The postoperative death rate has a provision that limits deaths to within 10 days of the surgery. Two reasons for this are the difficulty of locating patients more than 10 days after surgery, and also the possibility of a cause and effect relationship between the surgery and the death as the time from surgery increases.

 Calculating Postoperative Mortality Rates

$$\frac{\text{Total surgical deaths within 10 days postop}}{\text{Total surgical patients}} \times 100$$

Any deaths that are assigned to an anesthesia death rate must be done so on the death certificate. These rates are extremely small, usually around 1 in 100,000–250,000. Notice that it is not calculated by the number of discharges or by the number of surgical patients, because not all discharged patients have had an anesthetic agent administered, and surgical patients may have had more than one anesthetic agent administered.

 Calculating Anesthesia Death Rates

$$\frac{\text{Total deaths due to anesthesia}}{\text{Total number of times anesthesia was administered}} \times 100,000$$

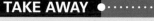

TAKE AWAY

Postoperative and anesthesia death rates give us more specific information about how surgical patients are dying in the hospital.

BRIEF CASE

COMPARING MORTALITY RATES

Michael looks at the national statistics for mortality rates for weight loss surgeries and compares them to mortality rates for other common surgeries at the hospital. He finds that the mortality rates are significantly smaller than some of the other types of surgeries.

Mortality rates following common operations in U.S. hospitals

	Heart bypass	Prostate	Esophageal resection	Hip replacement
National average mortality rate	3.5	0.5	9.1	0.3

Mortality rates following weight loss surgery

Gastric bypass	Sleeve gastrectomy	Gastric band
0.18% or 1 in 550	0.16% or 1 in 625	0.03% or 1 in 3,330

Continued

BRIEF CASE—cont'd

Next, Michael wonders if the data from his own hospital system would show similar results. Calculate the postop mortality rates for each of the following surgeries performed at Diamonte over the five years from 2011 to 2015, rounded to the thousandth place.

POSTOPERATIVE DEATHS BY PROCEDURE	2011	2012	2013	2014	2015	POSTOP MORTALITY RATE
Coronary artery bypass graft (CABG)	74	38	46	78	75	
Hip replacement	8	8	5	10	10	
Gastric bypass	4	11	5	0	0	
Sleeve gastrectomy	3	1	3	2	3	
Total surgeries performed	**1897**	**2232**	**2192**	**1898**	**1950**	

EXERCISE 5-4
Mortality Rates

1. Last year, your facility had 43 total deaths. Twenty-seven of the 43 total deaths occurred less than 48 hours after admission, and there were 6372 total discharges. Calculate gross and net mortality rates for your facility, rounded to two decimal places

2. In the month of July, there were 17 deaths reported that were within 10 days of surgery and 85 surgical patients. What was the postop death rate?

3. In the month of August, one death due to anesthetics of the 1011 anesthetics administered occurred. What is the anesthesia death rate per 100,000 people?

AUTOPSY RATES

An **autopsy** (also called a postmortem exam or necropsy) is an examination of the body after death to either determine or confirm the cause of death. The examination may be on the entire body or just part of it. Autopsies are not legally required unless the death is of an unnatural, suspicious, or unexpected nature, but they can serve as a quality measure to verify a clinical judgment for cause of death.

Hospital autopsies are requested by physicians or family members of the deceased for medical and/or educational purposes, while *medicolegal autopsies* are performed to investigate the cause of death. Hospital autopsies require the consent of the next of kin, while medicolegal autopsies do not. Not all families are willing to consent to an autopsy, and the responsibility for the request for autopsy usually rests with the attending physician. This is understandable; the request comes at a time when the family is grieving, and it has no effect on the outcome of treatment. Also, autopsies are expensive, ranging from $1500 to $5000, and they are seldom covered by external sources. So unless a family (or hospital) is willing to pay for the procedure, the cost for hospital autopsies is often prohibitive.

The rates that measure autopsies include or exclude certain types of patients, comparing the autopsies performed in the numerator to the number of corresponding deaths in the denominator. Like all rates, we are calculating a part (the type of patient: deceased inpatients, outpatients, former patients, newborns) of the whole (total

 Autopsy An examination of the body after death to either determine or confirm the cause of death.

TABLE 5-2

AUTOPSY RATES SUMMARY

TYPE OF AUTOPSY RATE	NUMERATOR	ADDITIONS/ SUBTRACTIONS FROM NUMERATOR	DENOMINATOR	ADDITIONS/ SUBTRACTIONS FROM DENOMINATOR
Gross	Total number of inpatient autopsies	——	Total number of inpatient deaths	——
Net	Total number of inpatient autopsies	——	Total number of inpatient deaths	Minus ME cases
Adjusted	Total number of inpatient autopsies	Plus non-inpatient hospital deaths (outpatients, former inpatients, hospice patients)	Total number of inpatient deaths	Minus ME cases Plus deaths of non-inpatient deaths used in numerator

inpatient deaths, total bodies available for autopsy, total newborn deaths). Table 5-2 summarizes the structure of the various types of autopsy formulas. So, if we want to know the *gross autopsy rate* for the inpatients in our hospital, what does the formula look like? The gross inpatient hospital autopsy rate includes only the autopsies done on a hospital's inpatient deaths for a given period of time.

 Calculating Gross Autopsy Rates

$$\frac{\text{Total number of autopsies performed on inpatients for a period}}{\text{Total number of inpatient deaths for this period}} \times 100$$

Stat Tip ···

Take note of the denominator in the above formula. Unlike the other rates we have looked at in this chapter, the whole is not total discharges, only inpatient deaths. Remember, we always calculate the rate by taking the number of occurrences and dividing it by the number of times it *could have happened*. Obviously, only deaths will be autopsied.

Additional criteria include the type of professional who performs the autopsy, and the facility where the autopsy is performed. The individual who performs the hospital autopsy (the hospital pathologist or another physician who has been assigned the duty) must be either on staff at that particular hospital or have been designated as the one who performs the autopsies for the hospital.

In the United States, the medicolegal autopsies are performed by one of three professionals: a coroner, a medical examiner (ME), or a forensic pathologist. Each state has its own system. American coroners are elected or appointed officials and do not necessarily have any medical background. MEs are physicians who are appointed and may or may not have advanced training and board certification in forensic pathology. Whether coroner, ME, or forensic pathologist, each position is responsible for ascertaining the cause of death. In the event of a natural death, the death certificate is signed by the patient's primary care giver (physician, physician assistant, or nurse practitioner, depending on the state). If an unexpected, unnatural death, the death certificate would be signed by the coroner, ME, or the forensic pathologist.

ME Medical examiner.

The physical location of the autopsy can be either at the hospital or at a location designated by the hospital for the purpose of having their autopsies performed. Large teaching hospitals may have their own pathology department that is the site of their autopsies, while a community hospital may have their pathologist use space off site from their own hospital. For the autopsy to be credited to the hospital, it must be performed by their own (or a designated) pathologist and in their own (or a designated) facility.

It is important to note that the hospital cannot perform an autopsy on an ME case (also called coroner's case) because the body is removed for legal reasons. In this case, there is no opportunity for the hospital to perform the autopsy, so the *net autopsy rate* corrects for that situation and does not "penalize" the hospital for not doing the autopsy.

 Calculating Net Autopsy Rates

$$\frac{\text{Total number of autopsies performed on inpatients for a period}}{\text{Total number of IP deaths} - \text{those bodies removed by MEs for this period}} \times 100$$

Not all autopsies performed at the hospital are strictly those of inpatients who died there; there may be former patients (those who had been discharged alive) as well. When calculating autopsy rates, inpatient hospital autopsies may be separated from total hospital autopsies, with the latter including bodies of these former patients. This is called the *adjusted (hospital) autopsy rate*. It includes those done on inpatients, subtracts the bodies of patients removed by the coroner or ME, and adds in the autopsies done on former patients (whether inpatient or outpatient).

 Calculating Adjusted (Hospital) Autopsy Rates

$$\frac{\begin{array}{c}\text{Total number of autopsies performed on inpatients}\\ +\ \text{autopsies on former patients}\\ -\ \text{bodies removed by the ME for a period}\end{array}}{\begin{array}{c}\text{Total number of IP deaths}\\ +\ \text{bodies of former patients available for autopsy}\\ -\ \text{those bodies removed by MEs for this period}\end{array}} \times 100$$

Here, the hospital has the best reflection of its actual work because it removes the cases that the hospital could not have performed autopsies on, and it includes the ones that are done on former patients. Former patients may be outpatients, home health care patients, same day surgery patients, hospice patients, or any other hospital patients who died and their bodies are available for autopsy.

You may note that if you calculate each of the rates in order from gross to net to adjusted, the rate gradually rises with the adjusted rate giving the most favorable percentage of autopsies. For example: Happy Valley Hospital reports 24 inpatient deaths in the month of March. Of those deaths, 6 are autopsied in the hospital, 1 is removed by the ME, and 2 bodies of former patients (one home health care patient and one outpatient) are returned to the hospital for autopsy. Below are the three autopsy rates, rounded to a whole number:

- Gross: $\dfrac{6}{24} \times 100 = 25\%$

- Net: $\dfrac{6}{24 - 1} \times 100 = 26\%$

- Adjusted: $\dfrac{6+2}{24+2-1} \times 100 = 32\%$

Notice the gross rate is the least, the net is second, and adjusted is the highest rate.

In 2012, the American Medical Association published a report expressing concern regarding the dwindling number of autopsies and the resulting effect on the reliability of our cause of death statistics.[2] In the article, the author cited a study from *Histopathology* in 2005 that found "half of autopsies produce medical findings that were unsuspected before the patient died." Another finding by a CDC study was that nearly one-third of all death certificates contain incorrect information for the cause of death.[3] Unfortunately, these inaccurate death certificates are filed with the National Center for Health Statistics and are compiled to give a national picture of the causes of death each year. How does this happen?

The Joint Commission (TJC), a voluntary health care accreditation organization, stopped requiring a minimal percentage of autopsies (20%) for hospital deaths in the 1970s, and the rate has continued to decline to the current day.[4] In addition, fewer older adult patients die in acute care hospitals, as DRG reimbursement rules encourage the transfer of elderly patients to skilled nursing and long-term care facilities, like nursing homes. As many as 33% of all elder adults now die in these settings, many of which do not have the resources to perform autopsies. A 2008 paper published in *Geriatrics* noted that the elderly have the lowest autopsy rate of any age group, citing the primary reason as "a supposed 'kindness' on the part of families and clinicians reluctant to inflict further 'discomfort' upon the deceased."[5] An article published by NCBI noted that families are more likely to give permission for autopsies of fetal, pediatric, and emergency department deaths.[6] Box 5-2 lists the specific formulas for these autopsy rates.

TJC The Joint Commission.

DRG Diagnosis-related group.

BOX 5-2   AUTOPSY FORMULAS

Formulas for fetal deaths, pediatric deaths, and emergency department deaths are as follows:

✎ **Calculating Fetal Death Autopsy Rates**

$$\frac{\text{Total number of autopsies performed on fetal deaths for a period}}{\text{Total number of fetal deaths for this period}} \times 100$$

✎ **Calculating Pediatric Autopsy Rates**

Note that you will need to consult your hospital for a definition of the range of ages for pediatric deaths.

$$\frac{\text{Total number of autopsies performed on pediatric deaths for a period}}{\text{Total number of pediatric deaths for this period}} \times 100$$

✎ **Calculating Emergency Department Autopsy Rates**

$$\frac{\text{Total number of autopsies performed on ED deaths for a period}}{\text{Total number of deaths occurring in the ED for this period}} \times 100$$

---

[2] http://www.amednews.com/article/20120220/health/302209940/4/.

[3] http://www.washingtonpost.com/blogs/wonkblog/wp/2013/05/12/study-nearly-half-of-all-death-certificates-are-wrong/.

[4] http://www.thedp.com/article/2012/02/autopsy_rate_at_hup_around_nation_on_the_decline.

[5] Libow, LS and Neufeld, RR. The autopsy and the elderly patient in the hospital and the nursing home: enhancing the quality of life. Geriatrics. December 2008; 63(12): 14–18.

[6] http://www.ncbi.nlm.nih.gov/pubmed/11418012.

BRIEF CASE

FINDING THE AUTOPSY RATE

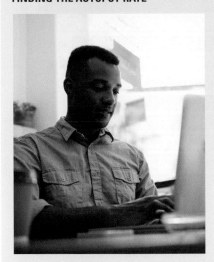

After lunch, Michael receives a request from the hospital administration. The COO is asking for autopsy rates throughout the enterprise over the last five years, noting that the Diamonte hospital system had acquired an academic medical center three years ago. Although Michael remembers studying these rates in school, he has not had a reason to use them until now. A quick check on the internet gives him an overview of some of the reasons why these statistics are so seldom requested (Fig. 5-5).

In short, he found that US autopsy rates had been declining for more than 50 years and the types of autopsies had changed proportionally during that time. The Joint Commission had dropped the requirement for a 20% autopsy rate in the 1970s, and the national rate had dwindled to about 8 to 9% currently. Autopsies for deaths due to diseases were low. The administrative request was a query to see if this finding was being reversed as a result of a policy change last year.

Looking at a graph from the NCHS (Fig. 5-6), Michael can see that the external causes of death (assaults, poisonings, and suicides, for example) comprised the majority of reasons for autopsy.

While the autopsies for external causes have been slowly rising, the total autopsies and those done to confirm causes of death due to disease were slowly sinking. A related graph (Fig. 5-7) showed that the autopsy rate for the elderly was very low (≥85 = 0.8%), while the rate for those in the 15–24 range was extremely high (60.3%).

Again, the causes of death for the young are almost always external, while those of the elderly are most often due to disease.

Michael flips open his text and reviews the formulas for the rates. He remembers that there were a couple tricky bits with definitions and adding and subtracting patients for the different rates.

● **COO** Chief operating officer.

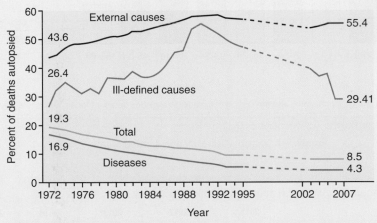

Notes: Includes data for 46 states and the District of Columbia (excludes data for Florida, Minnesota, New Mexico, and Pennsylvania). The 46 states and the District of Columbia accounted for 86 percent to 87 percent of all deaths in the United States. No data are available for 1995-2002 because the states did not provide that item to the National Center for Health Statistics for those years.
Source: CDC/NCHS, National Vital Statistics System, Mortality.

Figure 5-5 Trend in the autopsy rate: United States, 1972–2007.

BRIEF CASE—cont'd

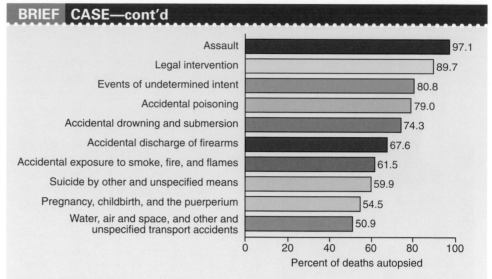

Notes: Includes data for 46 states and the District of Columbia (excludes data for Florida, Minnesota, New Mexico, and Pennsylvania). The 46 states and the District of Columbia accounted for 86 percent of all deaths.
Source: CDC/NCHS, National Vital Statistics System, Mortality.

Figure 5-6 Ten most common autopsied causes: United States, 2007.

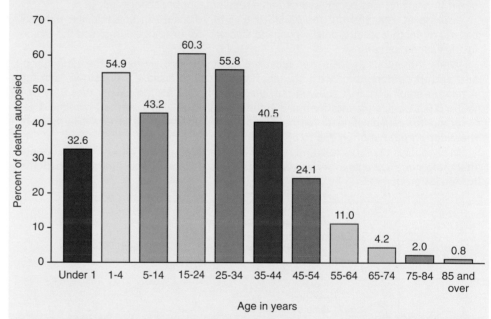

Notes: Includes data for 46 states and the District of Columbia (excludes data for Florida, Minnesota, New Mexico, and Pennsylvania). The 46 states and the District of Columbia accounted for 86 percent of all deaths.
Source: CDC/NCHS, National Vital Statistics System, Mortality.

Figure 5-7 Autopsy Rate, by age: United States, 2007.

Here is Michael's data before and after the acquisition of the academic hospital, St. Barnabas. Calculate the adjusted (hospital) autopsy rate for each year.

	2011	2012	2013[a]	2014	2015
IP deaths	143	179	223	301	316
IP autopsies	5	7	10	18	25
Autopsies on former patients	1	3	5	9	11
Bodies removed by MEs	3	1	4	9	8
Adjusted autopsy rate					

[a]Diamonte acquired St. Barnabas 11/30/2013.

EXERCISE 5-5

Autopsy Rates

Use the following year-end data to calculate the requested statistics. Round to the nearest whole number.

2 fetal autopsies

6 autopsies on pediatric patients

11 autopsies on emergency room patients

17 fetal deaths

13 pediatric deaths

126 emergency room deaths

1. Calculate the fetal autopsy rate.
2. Calculate the pediatric autopsy rate.
3. Calculate the emergency room autopsy rate.

REVIEW QUESTIONS

Refer to the data from St. Barnabas below, and use the appropriate formula in the chapter to calculate the following rates.

ST. BARNABAS HOSPITAL
SEPTEMBER 2016
400 beds, 15 bassinets

Admissions			Autopsies	
A&C	8612		**Hospital inpatients**	
Nb	365		A&C	11
Discharges			Nb	3
(including deaths)			**Hospital outpatients**	1
A&C	8589		**Home health patients**	3
Nb	361		**Fetal autopsies**	1
Obstetrical discharges	355		**ME cases**	5
(included in totals above)			**Fetal deaths**	
Pulmonary service	4		Early	2
discharges			Late	3
Deaths (total)			**Operations**	
	<48 hrs	>48 hrs	Total	2106
A&C	14	31	**Postoperative deaths**	28
Nb	2	1	(included in totals above)	
Postoperative deaths	28		**Anesthetics administered**	2099
(included in totals above)			**Deliveries**	
Deaths due to an anesthetic	1		Vaginal births	313
agent			CSs	42
Maternal Mortality			VBACs	4
Direct	2		**Infections**	
Indirect	5		Postoperative infections	3
Ventilator measures			Hospital infections	9
Ventilator days	34		**Consultations**	67
Patients with VAP	2			
Patients on ventilators	9			

1. Infection rate (round to two decimal places)

2. Postoperative infection rate (round to two decimal places)

3. VAP in ventilator usage rate (round to a whole number)

4. Consultation rate (round to a whole number)

5. MMR (round to two decimal places)

6. CS rate (round to one decimal place)

7. VBAC rate (round to one decimal place)

8. Early and late still birth rate (round to one decimal place)

9. Gross mortality rate (round to two decimal places)

10. Net mortality rate (round to two decimal places)

11. Anesthesia death rate (round to two decimal places)

12. Fetal autopsy rate (round to a whole number)

13. Gross autopsy rate (round to a whole number)

14. Net autopsy rate (round to a whole number)

15. Adjusted (hospital) autopsy rate (round to a whole number)

PUBLIC HEALTH DATA

CHAPTER OUTLINE

KEY TERMS

abortion rate
adjusted rate
confounding variable
crude rate
epidemiology
incidence

induced termination of pregnancy
   rate (ITOP)
mid-interval population
morbidity
mortality
natality

prevalence
public health statistics
specific rate
vital statistics

LEARNING OBJECTIVES

At the end of the chapter, you should be able to:
1. Define key terms.
2. List sources of public health data.
3. Differentiate among crude, specific, and adjusted rates.

4. Recognize and recall formulas for public health statistics.
5. Analyze sample public health data for various rates.

○ **Public health statistics** Statistics that describe the wellbeing of populations, such as an entire city, state, or country.

○ **Natality** Birth rate.

○ **Mortality** Death rate.

○ **Morbidity** A disease or illness.

○ **Vital statistics** Public health data collected through birth certificates, death certificates, and other data-gathering tools.

○ **NVSS** National Vital Statistics System.

○ **NCHS** National Center for Health Statistics.

I n the last chapter, we collected and analyzed data at the hospital level and physician practice level to track and trend activities within a facility, generating statistics to determine *how well* a particular facility was providing care. When statistics are used to convey information about the bigger picture—the wellbeing of populations of cities, counties, states, and countries—they are called **public health statistics**. Public health statistics show trends in a population. The statistics may describe factors related to **natality** (the birth rate) and **mortality** (the death rate), or they may be about **morbidity**—the diseases, disorders, and injuries that happen throughout a lifespan. Policymakers use public health statistics to plan and monitor public health initiatives, and hospitals and practice facilities may want to use these data to benchmark their data against national trends.

Morbidity statistics are collected by the Centers for Disease Control and Prevention (CDC) and provide valuable information about the occurrences of various diseases, disorders, and injuries in the United States. A special subset of public health statistics, called **vital statistics**, measures births, adoptions, deaths, marriages, and divorces in a population. The National Vital Statistics System (**NVSS**), within the National Center for Health Statistics (**NCHS**), is responsible for collecting and publishing reports that mainly measure the factors involved in growth or decline of the United States (US) population as a whole, and by race and ethnicity. For example, Figure 6-1 is a graph that shows the infamous baby boomer population increase after the Second World War. Knowing that this population is now reaching retirement age helps in planning for the large numbers of citizens who will need care for the disorders that affect an aging population, and planning for the expense that will result.

TAKE AWAY •••

Public health statistics measure trends in the health of populations. They are useful for planning and monitoring public health initiatives and providing comparative data for facilities.

BRIEF CASE

IDENTIFYING TRENDS

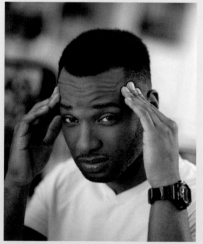

Michael hangs up the phone and rubs his temples. He now has numerous requests for data from departments across the system!

- The hospital has been experiencing a decreasing number of deliveries over the last few years, and the C-suite is asking for statistics on national trends to see if this is a local or national phenomenon.
- Social Services is asking for a comparison of their statistics to national trends for their teen pregnancy rates.
- The head of infectious disease wants information regarding measles incidence rates to see if his/her rates are aligned with national trends.

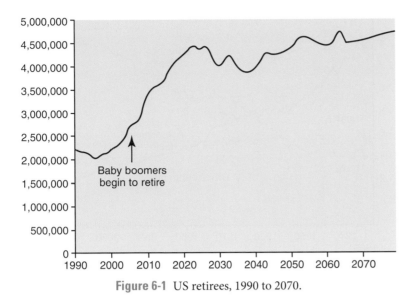

Figure 6-1 US retirees, 1990 to 2070.

TYPES OF RATES AND DIFFERENCES IN CONSTANTS

Public health statistics can be calculated in three different ways:

- **crude rates**, which compare the number of events to the entire population at risk
- **specific rates**, which compare the number of events within a given demographic (age, race, sex, etc.) to the population at risk
- **adjusted rates**, which compare the number of events observed to a *normalized* population.

A particular crude rate (for births or deaths) is calculated by comparing the number of events to the population at a given period of time and multiplying the result by 1000. Calculate population-specific rates by limiting analysis to certain ages, ethnic groups, or regions. Adjusted rates are by far the most complex, but are useful in comparing population statistics of two differently weighted populations. For example, you might compare birth rates among two states, North Dakota (16 births per 1000 people) and Pennsylvania (10 births per 1000). North Dakota has a much higher birth rate, but does this mean that people in North Dakota are more interested in having children than people in Pennsylvania? Not necessarily: we are comparing birth rates for a state that has a large elderly population (Pennsylvania) and a state that has a much younger population mix, that is, more people of childbearing age. If we do not "normalize" the populations, we may come to conclusions that are skewed by these differences. Using only crude birth rates would result in this type of error. In this case, the normalization of the population allows us to remove age, which is a **confounding variable**, a variable that masks the true findings.

Figure 6-2 shows how these types of rates compare and contrast. The graph compares the raw number of deaths, a crude death rate, and an adjusted death rate. Although the raw number of deaths appears to be dramatically increasing, the rates (actual numbers compared to the populations at risk) are in decline. On closer inspection, you will see that the age-adjusted rate is declining more rapidly than the crude rate. A walk-through of the steps to calculate adjusted rates is provided in the section on mortality.

While hospital statistics measure most of their rates in percentages, public health (including vital statistics) rates are usually expressed as per 1000, or sometimes more. The reason for the difference is that the use of a larger constant results in a whole number of persons. This allows us to visualize a birth, death, or disease rate of, for example, three people per 1000—instead of 0.3 per 100.

Crude rate A rate comparing the number of events (births, deaths, diseases, etc.) to the entire population at risk for the event.

Specific rate A rate comparing the number of events (births, deaths, diseases, etc.) within a demographic subset of a population (people of a certain age, race, sex, etc.) to the entire population at risk for the event.

Adjusted rate A rate comparing the number of events (births, deaths, diseases, etc.) among populations with different demographic makeups (such as age, race, or gender) as if the two populations had the same makeup.

Confounding variable An extra factor that masks the real relationship of occurrence or event to the population at risk for the event.

TAKE AWAY

Data analysts may want to adjust the populations of two groups by age, comparing the two populations as if there were the same number of people in each age group.

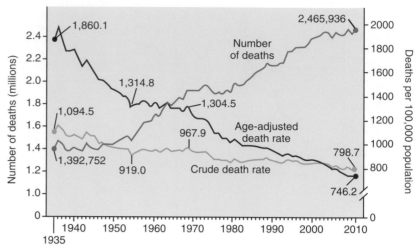

Figure 6-2 Number of deaths, crude and age-adjusted death rates: United States, 1935 to 2010.

To compare public health rates, you must locate a population estimate for the particular group in question. The NCHS uses census and *intercensal* data—an estimation of population between regular censuses—for their comparisons. These population estimates can be stated as the "mid-interval" population or the "mean" population. What is the difference? The **mid-interval population** is a measure of the population at the midpoint of the time interval, whether that is a month, a year, or longer. The mean population is an average of the collection periods (for example, the average of the months during a given year). Mean population data are more often used in areas where there are large population changes throughout the period being measured, such as a seasonal change due to climate. The United States uses the mid-interval measure for their data provided by NCHS, and all of our formulas that use a denominator of total population are using a mid-interval population.

> ⭕ **Mid-interval population** The size of the population at the midpoint of a period of time.

⋮ EXERCISE 6-1

⋮ Types of Rates and Differences in Constants

1. Public health statistics show _____ in a population.

2. List four life events measured by vital statistics, a subset of public health statistics.

3. Public health statistics measure trends and are useful as _____ data for facilities.

4. The National Vital Statistics System (NVSS) is part of which government agency?

5. Natality data measures factors regarding _____.

6. Data regarding diseases, disorders, and injuries are _____ data.

7. Data regarding causes of death are _____ data.

8. What type of rate allows the health data analyst to remove a confounding variable?

BOX 6-1	SUMMARY OF NATALITY STATISTICS, UNITED STATES, FINAL DATA FOR 2012

- Number of births: 3,952,841
- Birth rate: 12.6 per 1000 population
- Fertility rate: 63.0 births per 1000 women aged 15 to 44 years
- Percent born low birth weight: 8.0%
- Percent born preterm: 11.5%
- Percent unmarried: 40.7%
- Mean age at first birth: 25.8

From Births: Final Data for 2012 by Joyce A. Martin, M.P.H.; Brady E. Hamilton, Ph.D.; Michelle J.K. Osterman, M.H.S.; Sally C. Curtin, M.A. and T.J. Mathews, M.S., Division of Vital Statistics, http://www.cdc.gov/nchs/data/nvsr/nvsr62/nvsr62_09.pdf.

NATALITY DATA

The legal responsibility for the registration of births (and deaths, marriages, and divorces) resides with each state. Although the reporting of the statistics by each state is mandatory, the format for reporting is not. In 2003, **NVSS** published a set of birth (and death) certificates, but the use of these forms is a guideline, not a mandate. The current projection for a standardized reporting system of birth certificates is in 2015.

NVSS National Vital Statistics System.

The NVSS collects the information from the state registration sites and publishes the findings in a number of reports including Health E-Stats, National Vital Statistics Report (NVSR), and Data Briefs. Box 6-1 is a summary of some of the NVSS results from 2012, showing the vital statistics routinely collected for natality: a count of births, a rate per 1000, a fertility rate, preterm and low birth weight percentages, average age of mother at first birth, and the percentage of births to unmarried women. To give greater context to any of these, they can also be viewed as part of a trend, broken down by a number of different factors, and viewed by state as well.

We will look at the calculation and examples of these natality rates below, but it is worth noting that this is just a sampling of the information that can be drawn from vital statistics—there are many more rates used for research, planning, and benchmarking. For example, it is interesting to know that births to unmarried women have climbed to almost 41%. But when we narrow the calculations further by age groups, we find that these births are not to teenagers but to women in their twenties or older. Teenagers account for only 23% of out-of-wedlock births. As you can see, the public health data provide valuable information about trends in the overall population.

Birth and Obstetrical Rate Formulas

Crude Birth Rate

Birth rates are expressed as "births per 1000 people" to make them comparable between different communities. This is a measure of how fast a population is growing. Calculate crude birth rates by dividing the total number of live births (for the population of interest) over a 1 year period by the total mid-interval population during that year, then multiplying by 1000.

 Calculating the Crude Birth Rate

$$\frac{\text{Number of live births in a given period}}{\text{Mid - interval population in that period}} \times 1000$$

For example, let us say that Stark County begins with a population of 50,000 in January 2015 and ends with an estimated 50,500 people. Stark County's mid-interval population estimate on July 1st is 50,250 people. During 2014, they counted 738 live births. We calculate the crude birth rate for Stark County in 2015 as follows:

$$\frac{738}{50,250} \times 1000 = 14.69 \text{ live births per thousand}$$

Fertility Rate

You might have noticed that the crude rate does not take into account the sex of the population; that is, the denominator includes both men and women. A more accurate indication of the birth rate in a community, state, or the nation would remove males and focus the denominator, the number of times something *could happen*, on the number of women of childbearing age.

Calculate fertility rates by dividing the total number of births over a 1 year period by the total population of women ages 15 to 44 during that year (the age range used by the National Center for Healthcare Statistics), then multiplying by 1000. Fertility rates are expressed as "births per 1000 women" to make them comparable between different communities. This rate is used to evaluate how many children, on average, are born to women in a community.

 Calculating the Fertility Rate

$$\frac{\text{Number of live births in a given period}}{\text{Population of females from ages 15 to 44}} \times 1000$$

If Stark County reported 16,085 women aged 15 to 44 midyear in 2015, the fertility rate is calculated as

$$\frac{738}{16,085} \times 1000 = 45.88 \text{ live births per 1000 women ages 15 to 44.}$$

Miscellaneous Birth Rates

Some rates can tell us about the societal trends in a population. For example, calculating the number of children born out of wedlock might give us insight into demographic shifts in the population; calculating the teenage pregnancy ratio could tell us about the efficacy of sex education programs.

 Calculating the Out-of-Wedlock Birth Ratio

$$\frac{\text{Out-of-wedlock live births}}{\text{Mid-interval population}} \times 1000$$

 Calculating the Teenage Pregnancy Rate

$$\frac{\text{Number of live births among females ages 15 to 19}}{\text{Mid-interval female population from the same ages}} \times 1000$$

Stat Tip ···

It is interesting to note that if the birth is reported in pounds and ounces instead of grams, the reporting directions for the uniform birth certificate ask that the conversion *not* be done.

BRIEF CASE

BENCHMARKING AGAINST NATIONAL RATES

Michael wants to look in to the reduced delivery rates at the hospital and compare his trend data to the national figures. He locates a copy of the ICD-9-CM code for normal deliveries from 1993 to 2012 at HCUPnet (hcupnet.ahrq.gov). To use HCUPnet, he chooses "National Statistics on All Stays," identifies himself as a "researcher, medical professional," chooses the option for "Trends," chooses "specific diagnosis by ICD-9-CM," chooses "principal diagnosis," locates the correct ICD-9-CM diagnosis, chooses "number of discharges," and asks for a graph of his results:

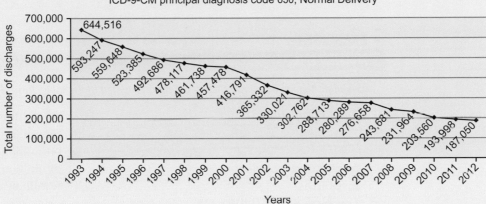

Total number of discharges
ICD-9-CM principal diagnosis code 650, Normal Delivery

He also pulls up a chart from the NVSS for out-of-hospital birth rates from 1990 to 2012. He can clearly see the trend of diminishing *hospital* births nationally.

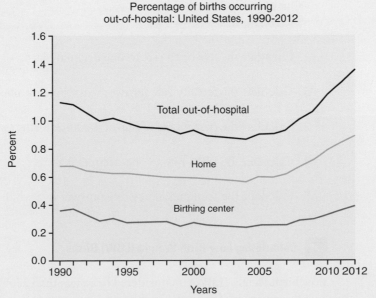

Percentage of births occurring
out-of-hospital: United States, 1990-2012

Note: Out-of-hospital births include those occurring in a home, birthing center, clinic or doctor's office, or other location.
Source: CDC/NCHS, National Vital Statistics System, birth certificate data.

Continued

BRIEF CASE—cont'd

After he finds one more measure that showed an uptick in the number of out of hospital births, he pastes the charts, tables, and sources into a file for a report that he will work on later in the day. He makes a note to check the formulas for the hospital birth rate and public health birth rates.

Maybe the trend for having babies outside of a hospital setting, either at home or in a birthing center, along with a diminishing national birth rate, might have something to do with the statistics?

Next, he wants to provide some data for the Teen and Pregnant Program on the efficacy of its awareness initiatives. He locates the hospital's stats for teen pregnancy for the past three years.

Year	Teenage Birth Rate
2011	26.1/1000
2012	23.9/1000
2013	19.4/1000

He wants to compare them to the NVSS ages 15 to 19 birth rates for all races and origins in his report.

Using the Website listed, find the national rates for 2011, 2012, and 2013 and in Excel, plot them against Michael's hospital statistics (refer to http://www.cdc.gov/nchs/data/nvsr/nvsr64/nvsr64_01.pdf).

EXERCISE 6-2

Natality Data

Calculate the following rates using the data provided in the table. Round as indicated.

Total Population	300 million
Women	152 million
Men	148 million
Mid-interval population	300 million
Live births	4 million
Low birth weight (LBW)	300,000
Teenage mid-interval population (women 15-19)	11,000,000
Teenage live births	350,000
Out of wedlock births	1,600,000
Live births to women 15-44	3,900,000

1. Calculate the live birth rate to one decimal place.

2. Calculate the fertility rate (answer in a whole number).

3. Calculate the percentage of out-of-wedlock births (whole percentage).

4. Calculate the LBW rate to one decimal place.

5. Calculate the teen pregnancy rate (answer in a whole number).

Calculating Low Birth Weight (LBW) Births

Low birth weight (LBW) is considered to be less than 2500 g (about 5 pounds 8 ounces) and is a measure of neonatal health.

$$\frac{\text{Number of low birth weight (LBW) babies}}{\text{Total live births}} \times 1000$$

MORTALITY STATISTICS

We can be very general (crude) when calculating mortality rates in a population, or we can be more specific. Although it might be interesting that, in a particular state last year, there were a total of 6 deaths for every 1000 people, it is probably more helpful to know rates by age, ethnicity, gender, race, or cause. Do Hispanics die at a higher rate than non-Hispanics? Do men die at a higher rate than women? What is the rate for people under 24? What are the causes of death?

Who, when, and how people within a population die vary based on a number of factors. The leading causes of death are different depending on one's age, sex, race, or location. In Figure 6-3, data from the World Health Organization (**WHO**) shows the causes of death for high- and low-income countries. Do you notice any trends? Many deaths in the higher income countries are lifestyle diseases, attributable to diet or smoking habits, while the lower income countries have more deaths resulting from communicable diseases.

As with birth certificates, a specific death certificate suggested by the **NVSS** cannot be mandated. As a result, the data will not be uniformly collected but are still

WHO World Health Organization.

TAKE AWAY ● · · · · · · · · · ·

Who, when, and how people within a population die vary based on a number of factors.

NVSS National Vital Statistics System.

High income

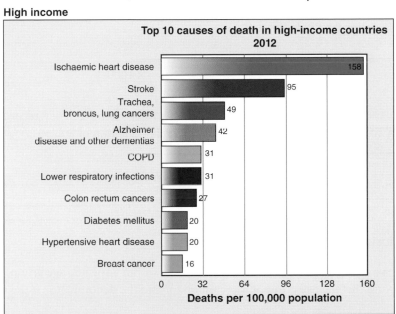

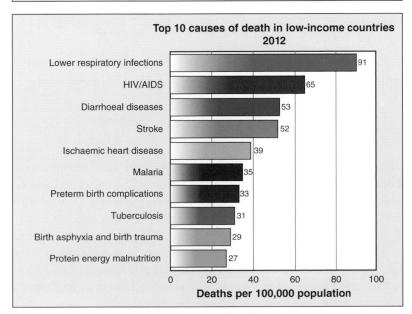

Figure 6-3 Mortality in low- and high-income countries.

reasonably reliable. The upper right-hand corner of the suggested model death certificate has a block for the Social Security Number of the decedent. This allows the death to be recorded in the Social Security Death Master File, used to verify reported deaths. A birth/death link registry (www.cdc.gov/nchs/linked.htm) is also useful for tracking trends regarding infant mortality. This registry links the birth certificate data (such as the ages and races of the baby's parents, birth weight, length of gestation, and more) for every infant under one year of age to the information on that child's death certificate, such as cause of death. Researcher can use the data set to explore how variables present during the development and birth of the fetus may contribute to infant death.

Mortality Rate Formulas

There are several formulas that measure death, many of them concerning obstetric-related causes. Each of the rates listed below tells us a different story about who is dying, when, and from what cause.

 Calculating the Crude Death Rate

$$\frac{\text{Total number of deaths}}{\text{Mid - interval population}} \times 1000$$

Let us use the same numbers for Stark County as an example. They recorded 1001 deaths in 2015 and have an estimated mid-interval population of 50,250.

$$\frac{1001}{50,250} \times 1000 = 19.92 \text{ deaths per thousand people}$$

 Calculating the Age-Specific Death Rate

Since we are only looking for the mortality rate within a specific age group, we need to make sure that the age group in the numerator and the denominator is the same.

$$\frac{\text{Total deaths in a specific age group}}{\text{Mid - interval population of the same age group}} \times 1000$$

Of the 1001 deaths in the county, 236 were among people ages 75 to 84. The mid-interval estimate on July 1st counts 2000 people ages 75 to 84 in the county.

$$\frac{236}{2000} \times 1000 = 118 \text{ deaths per thousand}$$

Certainly, physicians, researchers, and policymakers alike are interested in the causes of death in a population. Mortality rates for specific diseases and procedures can serve as rough quality measures, giving the individual physicians (and administrators) summaries of the outcomes of treatments. For example, CMS publicly reports 30-day mortality measures for heart failure, acute myocardial infarctions, and pneumonia. By using the individual ICD-10 codes for the variations in each of these (e.g., variations of pneumonia include B05.2, measles pneumonia; B59, pneumonia due to *Pneumocystis carinii*; or A02.22, *Salmonella pneumonia*), an analyst can target each of these cases and collect information that can be useful in lowering the rates.

Box 6-2 lists the leading causes of death in the US and the frequency of each in 2010.

- Heart disease: 596,577
- Cancer: 576,691
- Chronic lower respiratory diseases: 142,943
- Stroke (cerebrovascular diseases): 128,932
- Accidents (unintentional injuries): 126,438
- Alzheimer's disease: 84,974
- Diabetes: 73,831
- Influenza and pneumonia: 53,826
- Nephritis, nephrotic syndrome, and nephrosis: 45,591
- Intentional self-harm (suicide): 39,518

From Deaths: Final Data for 2011, Table 10, http://www.cdc.gov/nchs/data/nvsr63/nvsr63_03.pdf.

While the box provides the totals for the causes of deaths in 2010, it does not present them as a rate. If you wanted to see if the death rates for these causes were similar (or different) to your particular state, you would need to calculate a rate. The formula for this calculation is as follows:

 Calculating the Cause-Specific Death Rate

$$\frac{\text{Deaths due to a specific cause}}{\text{Mid-interval population for a given period}} \times 100,000$$

So, using the mid-interval census figure of 309,349,689,[1] the cause-specific death rate for heart disease would be

$$\frac{596,577}{309,349,689} \times 100,000 = 192.8 \text{ or } 193 \text{ deaths per } 100,000$$

The death rate for Alzheimer's disease in the US for 2010 would be $84,974 \times 100,000/309,349,689 = 27.4$ or 27 deaths per 100,000 population.

Stat Tip

Since 1999, the causes of death have been recorded using ICD-10 diagnoses. Researchers who want to dig back to find comparison data that were coded using ICD-9 will find that a bit more work is required. Viral hepatitis, for example, coded with ICD 9, is 070. In ICD-10, the codes are B15-B19. As always, a careful look will be required to compare similar diagnoses.

Age-Adjusted Death Rate

Adjusted rates, as we noted earlier, are used to standardize (or normalize) a population that has a skewed distribution of its population. For example, the state of Florida has a population that is proportionately older than average compared to the other states. Conversely, Utah has a younger population than other states. When trying to compare mortality rates in these two states to the national averages, it might appear as though

---

[1] 309,349,689 is the intercensal figure from http://www.census.gov/popest/data/intercensal/national/nat2010.html, and lists the date of the estimate as July 1, 2010.

MATH REVIEW

To gain a better sense of why this is important, it may be useful to reflect back on the influence of extreme values in a distribution and how they can influence the mean.

Florida were a more dangerous place to live or that its medical care was lacking in quality. If a state has a very high death rate and it is partially due to its population being older, a data analyst may want to adjust the population mortality figures to obtain a truer picture of who is dying in a particular population. We do this by comparing these rates to what they would look like if its populations were similar in composition to the national norms.

Statistical adjustment is a method that can be used to compare differently weighted populations. Adjustment is frequently done for age, but the concepts can also be applied to other variables, such as gender or race. Think about the following exam results that two students, Josh and Alex, receive in a health information course.

	# MC Q Correct		MC Q Weight		MC Total Points		# Essay Q Correct		Essay Q Weight		Essay Total Points		Exam Grade
Alex	0	×	3	=	0		10	×	7	=	70		70
Josh	10	×	3	=	30		0	×	7	=	0		30
	Correct Questions						**Total Points**						
Alex	10						70						
Josh	10						30						

The exam was composed of 10 multiple choice and 10 essay questions. Josh aced the multiple choice questions but got none of the essay questions correct. Alex got none of the multiple choice, but all of the essay questions correct. When the exams were handed back, Josh's grade was 70, while Alex got a 30. You might think that they should have each gotten the same grade, since they each answered 10 questions correctly. Instead, the multiple choice questions were worth only 3 points each, while the essay questions were worth 7 points each. Because of the way the questions were weighted, the grades ended up being very different.

Every 10 years, the US conducts a population census in which the age, gender, race, and many other variables of US citizens are collected. Those results are available through the Census Bureau (http://www.census.gov/) and provide a baseline of the population proportions that are "normal" for the 2010 census. By normal, we mean that these are the population proportions seen for the entire US population. While crude rates compare a variable to an entire population, age-adjusted rates allow you to compare one state to another (or a city to a state) by "removing" the influence of extremes in a particular population composition. The proportions are the weights that are used to equalize our comparisons. Using the example above, Josh and Alex could be different states with similar mortality rates (number of questions correct out of the total 10/20 = 50) but very differently weighted populations ($3 \times 10 = 30$ vs $7 \times 10 = 70$). In other words, by making different age segments of a population count more than others (i.e., assigning weights), we are able to truly compare populations with very different kinds of people.

The following example uses 2010 US Census data for the state with the lowest median age (Utah, with a median age of 29.2 years old) compared to one of the states with one of the oldest median ages (Pennsylvania, whose median age is 40.1 years old). Figure 6-4 shows the percentage of each state's population in each age range. Do you see how much larger the younger age ranges are for Utah compared to Pennsylvania? And how much older Pennsylvania is? Those differences give differing weights to whatever variable is attached, for example, the mortality of those age ranges. By adjusting (also called standardizing or normalizing) the population, you can get a better idea of the real effect of the variable (in this case, the number of deaths) without the different weighting of a state (for example) from the weighting of the nation.

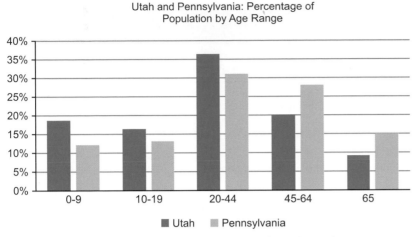

Figure 6-4 Utah and Pennsylvania: Percentage of population by age range.

The age ranges, crude death rate, and population proportions are provided for our standard population (the US) and the two populations of interest that we wish to compare with adjusted rates.

| | UTAH | | | |
Age Range	Population	Population Proportion	Deaths	Crude Death Rate (Out of 100,000)
0-9	513,496	0.18578776	334	12.08443911
10-19	449,041	0.16246732	138	4.992971849
20-44	1,004,681	0.36350318	1208	43.70659416
45-64	547,205	0.197984	2657	96.13279858
65+	249,462	0.09025774	10,439	377.6929937
Total	**2,763,885**		**14,776**	**534.6097974**
Pennsylvania				
0-9	1,483,173	0.1167634	1237	83.40227337
10-19	1,696,217	0.13353538	576	38.83565842
20-44	4,000,934	0.31497517	5333	133.2938759
45-64	3,562,748	0.2804788	21,547	604.7859686
65+	1,959,307	0.15424725	95,892	4894.179422
Not stated			11	
Total	**12,702,379**		**124,596**	**980.8871236**
United States				
0-9	40,550,019	0.13133799	31,232	77.0209257
10-9	42,717,537	0.13835839	13,836	32.3895079
20-44	103,720,553	0.33594187	130,956	126.258486
45-64	81,489,445	0.26393724	494,009	606.224524
65+	40,267,984	0.13042451	1,798,276	4465.77112
Total	**308,745,538**		**2,468,309**	**799.463861**

The crude and age-specific mortality rates by age distribution for Utah and Pennsylvania are not the same. While Pennsylvania has more deaths within each segment of the age ranges (it is a much more populous state), the rates are different depending on the age range.

Two different methods for adjusting the populations under scrutiny are called *direct adjustment* and *indirect adjustment*. *Direct adjustment* uses the mortality rates

TABLE 6-1

SUMMARY OF ADJUSTED RATES

TYPE OF ADJUSTED RATE/FEATURES	DIRECT ADJUSTMENT	INDIRECT ADJUSTMENT
Method	Proportion of US Pop (standard population) for each grouping × mortality rate for same grouping for state (population of interest)	Proportion of state population (population of interest) × mortality rate for US Pop (standard population) for same age groupings
Mortality rates used	Mortality rate for population of interest	Mortality rate for standard population
Proportions used	Proportion of standard population	Proportion of population of interest
Result	Standardized mortality rate for grouping	Expected mortality rate for grouping
Sum	Sum of all segments is the standardized mortality rate for population of interest	Sum of all segments is the expected death rate for the population of interest
Other derived rates	—	The standard mortality rate (SMR) is the ratio of observed death rate (actual deaths/state Pop of state × 100) divided by the expected death rate

of the population you wish to examine (for example, a state or city), while *indirect adjustment* uses the mortality rate of the standard population (in our example, the US, or it could be a state if you are examining a city). Indirect adjustment is used when the number of cases is small in the population under study or the data in question are not available as age-specific rates. Table 6-1 provides a summary of the two adjustment methods. It is important to remember that any differences that may be uncovered are due to the weighting of the death rates (or morbidity) in the population under scrutiny and are not actual findings. Adjusted rates are an extrapolation of what the expected figures *would be* if the weighting was the same as the standard population. A greater proportion of deaths in one age grouping of the population will change the overall standardized mortality rate because of the weight of those deaths in that segment.

 Calculating the Age-Adjusted Death Rate—Direct Method

You will need:
- The same age groupings for the standard population (our example uses the US population) and the observed population (in our example, the state population)
- The proportions for each of the standard population groupings
- The mortality rates for each of the standard population groupings
- The proportions for each of the observed population groupings
- The mortality rate for each of the observed population groupings

Stat Tip ··

Locate the Mortality Rates for your state or municipality through the Wonder CDC database at http://wonder.cdc.gov/cmf-icd10.html.

1. Multiply each of the US population groupings times the mortality rate for the same grouping of the state you are interested in examining.
2. The results will be the directly standardized mortality rates for each grouping, and the total of the rates will be the state age-adjusted mortality rate.
3. The sum of each of these will be the age-adjusted rate for the state population.
   Let us calculate the age-adjusted mortality rates for Utah and Pennsylvania using the direct method as an example.

UTAH

Age Range	Standard Population (US Population Proportion)	Mortality Rate of Population of Interest (Utah Crude Mortality Rate/100,000)	Estimated Mortality Rate for the Population of Interest
0-9	0.13	65	$65 \times 0.13 = 8.45$ or 8 per 100,000
10-19	0.14	31	$31 \times 0.14 = 4.34$ or 4 per 100,000
20-44	0.34	120	$120 \times 0.34 = 40.8$ or 41 per 100,000
45-64	0.26	486	$486 \times 0.26 = 126.36$ or 126 per 100,000
65+	0.13	4185	$4185 \times 0.13 = 544.05$ or 544 per 100,000

PENNSYLVANIA

Age Range	Standard Population (US Population Proportion)	Mortality Rate of Population of Interest (Pennsylvania Crude Mortality Rate/100,000)	Estimated Mortality Rate for the Population of Interest
0-9	0.13	83	$83 \times 0.13 = 10.79$ or 11 per 100,000
10-19	0.14	39	$39 \times 0.14 = 5.46$ or 5 per 100,000
20-44	0.34	133	$133 \times 0.34 = 45.22$ or 45 per 100,000
45-64	0.26	604	$604 \times 0.26 = 157.04$ or 157 per 100,000
65+	0.13	4894	$4894 \times 0.13 = 116.22$ or 116 per 100,000

By comparing the two sets of results, you can see that indeed, Pennsylvania does have a higher death rate *except* for the most elderly age range, where a directly adjusted rate reveals only 116 per 100,000 dying, as opposed to Utah's rate of 544 per 100,000.

 Calculating the Age-Adjusted Death Rate—Indirect Method

You will need:
- The same age groupings for the US population and the state population
- The proportions of the state population for those age groupings
- The US mortality rate for each of the age groupings

1. Multiply the deaths for each age grouping of the state population times the mortality rate for the same grouping of the US population.
2. The results will be the expected death rate for that proportion of the population.
3. The sum of each of these will add up to the expected death rate for the state.
4. The standard mortality rate (SMR) is the ratio of the observed death rate (the observed deaths $\times$ 100 $\div$ the population of the state) to the expected deaths $\times$ 100 $\div$ the population of the state.
5. If this ratio, multiplied by 100, is greater than the standard mortality rate, then the death rate is greater than expected. Conversely, if it is less than the SMR, the death rate is less than expected. *Remember these are not actual deaths, but an interpretation of the findings!*

Using an indirect method of adjustment, we again use population proportions and mortality rates, but switch the standard and population of interest for each. The indirect rate uses the proportions of the population of interest (here we will use Utah and Pennsylvania) and multiplies them by the standard (US) mortality rate for each corresponding age range.

UTAH

A	B	C	D (B×C)
Age Range	Utah Population Proportion	US Mortality Rate/100,000	Expected Deaths
0-9	0.19	77	14.63 rounded to 15
10-19	0.16	32	5.12 rounded to 5
20-44	0.36	126	45.36 rounded to 45
45-64	0.20	606	121.2 rounded to 121
65+	0.09	4466	401.9 rounded to 402

PENNSYLVANIA

A	B	C	D (B×C)
Age Range	PA Population Proportion	US Mortality Rate/100,000	Expected Deaths
0-9	0.12	77	9.24 rounded to 9
10-19	0.13	32	4.16 rounded to 4
20-44	0.31	126	39.06 rounded to 39
45-64	0.28	606	169.6 rounded to 170
65+	0.15	4466	669.9 rounded to 670

If the indirect adjusted rate is higher than the crude rate, it would mean that the expected mortality rate is greater than the standard population. However, if it is lower than the crude rate, your population being studied has a lower than expected mortality rate.

Maternal, Fetal, and Infant Mortality

Maternal mortality rates, along with mortality rates for fetuses, neonates, and infants, began to improve substantially in the middle of the twentieth century in the US and other developed countries. While each hospital will keep track of its own rates, NVSS keeps track of US national rates for these. It is important to note the large constants used for these formulas and the reasons why. Maternal mortality (with a constant of 100,000) is so exceedingly rare, that to put a "face" on this number, it is necessary to multiply by such a large constant to result in whole numbers. Neonatal mortality also requires a large constant, however, in this case, one of 10,000. This is because there are more neonates dying than mothers. Fetal deaths are the most common of these three obstetric-related mortality rates, recorded with a constant of 1000.

Maternal Mortality Rate

The CDC defines a pregnancy-related death as "the death of a woman during pregnancy or within one year of the end of pregnancy from a pregnancy complication, a chain of events initiated by pregnancy, or the aggravation of an unrelated condition by the physiologic effects of pregnancy."[2] A recent report shows that the US maternal mortality rate is trending back upward. Whether it is because maternal age is increasing or because of other health factors, it is a disturbing increase. Hospitals may want to benchmark their own statistics against the national trend to see how they are doing.

One way of thinking about maternal mortality is to count the number of maternal deaths and compare that number to the number of live births. While this formula leaves out the number of women who died before giving birth from the denominator, it gives a rough measure of mortality related to the outcome of live births.

 Calculating Maternal Mortality Rate

$$\frac{\text{Total maternal deaths}}{\text{Total live births}} \times 100,000$$

As an example, let us say hypothetically that a given state counted 18 maternal deaths within one year of the end of pregnancy from a pregnancy complication on its death certificates. That year, the state counted 143,514 live births.

$$\frac{18}{143,514} \times 100,000 = 12.57 \text{ maternal deaths per } 100,000 \text{ births}$$

Stat Tip ··

Remember that if you are comparing statistics, you will need to use the same formula as the statistic you are comparing—so check ahead of time for the previous formula used.

Abortion Rate

Also called the **induced termination of pregnancy (ITOP) rate**, the **abortion rate** is measured in two different ways: either comparing the number of legally induced abortions to the number of live births or comparing the same numerator to the population of women aged 15 to 44. Do not confuse *spontaneous abortions* (miscarriages or fetal deaths) with abortions. Nationally, in 2010, 765,651 legally induced abortions were reported to CDC. The abortion rate for 2010 was 14.6 abortions per 1000 women 15 to 44 years of age, and the abortion ratio was 228 abortions per 1000 live births.[3]

○ **Induced termination of pregnancy (ITOP) rate** The rate of legally induced abortions within a population. Also called the abortion rate.

○ **Abortion rate** The rate of legally induced abortions within a population. Also called the induced termination of pregnancy (ITOP) rate.

 Calculating the Abortion Rate—Method 1

$$\frac{\text{Legally induced abortions}}{\text{Mid-interval population of women aged 15 to 44}} \times 1000$$

---

[2] http://www.cdc.gov/reproductivehealth/MaternalInfantHealth/Pregnancy-relatedMortality.htm.
[3] http://www.cdc.gov/reproductivehealth/data_stats/.

TABLE 6-2	
FETAL AND NEONATAL AGE RANGES	
RATE	**AGE RANGE**
Miscarriage	<20 weeks' gestation
Early fetal	20-27 weeks' gestation
Late fetal	≥28 weeks' gestation
Perinatal	≥28 weeks' gestation to 8 days after birth
Neonatal	Birth to less than 28 days
Early neonatal	Birth to less than 7 days
Postnatal mortality rate	28 days to 1 year
Infant	Birth to 1 year

Calculating the Abortion Rate—Method 2

$$\frac{\text{Legally induced abortions}}{\text{Total live births}} \times 1000$$

Let us use some hypothetical numbers and plug them into each formula. In 2012, 11,674 induced abortions were recorded in the state. The state counted 49,211 births and a mid-interval population of women ages 15 to 44 of 745,313.

$$\frac{11,674}{745,313} \times 1000 = 15.66 \text{ abortions per 1000 females aged 15 to 44}$$

$$\frac{11,674}{49,211} \times 1000 = 237 \text{ abortions per 1000 live births}$$

Fetal and Neonatal Mortality Rates

As discussed in Chapter 5, the definition of a fetal death varies from state to state and may include the age of the fetus and the weight. "Early" fetal deaths are normally categorized from 20 to 27 weeks and "late" fetal deaths as 28 weeks or later, but again, check with your own state's definitions. A summary of the age periods used for each of the fetal and neonatal mortality rate calculations can be found in Table 6-2, and the formulas are presented below.

Calculating the Late Fetal Mortality Rate

$$\frac{\text{Number of late fetal deaths}}{\text{Live births} + \text{late fetal deaths (stillbirths)}} \times 1000$$

Calculating the Early Neonatal Mortality Rate

Early neonatal deaths are those that occur between birth and less than 7 days of life.

$$\frac{\text{Number of early neonatal (birth to <7 days) deaths}}{\text{Live births}} \times 1000$$

Calculating the Neonatal Mortality Rate

Neonatal deaths include deaths of infants between birth and the first 28 days of life.

$$\frac{\text{Number of newborn deaths ages birth to less than 28 days}}{\text{Live births}} \times 1000$$

 Calculating the Postnatal Mortality Rate

Postnatal mortality rates include deaths of infants after the neonatal period up to 1 year of life.

$$\frac{\text{Number of infant deaths from 28 days to 1 year}}{\text{Live births}} \times 1000$$

 Calculating the Perinatal Mortality Rate

Perinatal deaths are those that include both early and late fetal, and early neonatal deaths. They are compared to live births and late fetal deaths. Remember that all of these formulas compare what actually happened to what potentially could have happened—the fetal deaths could have been live births and need to be added to the live births to give the potential of possible births.

$$\frac{\text{Number of early and late fetal deaths} + \text{ early neonatal deaths}}{\text{Live births} + \text{ late fetal deaths}} \times 1000$$

 Calculating the Infant Mortality Rate

The infant mortality rate includes deaths of infants from birth through the first year of life.

$$\frac{\text{Number of infant deaths birth to 1 year}}{\text{Live births}} \times 1000$$

Take a look at the table below from the **NVSS**. Note that the combined early and late fetal and early neonatal mortality rates equal a perinatal mortality rate. It is also interesting to note that the early neonatal mortality rate is higher than the late fetal mortality rate. Could it be because of possible birth trauma?

NVSS National Vital Statistics System.

	FETAL DEATHS			INFANT DEATHS			
Year	Total*	20-27 Weeks	28 Weeks or More	Less Than 7 Days	Less Than 28 Days	Peri-natal Deaths	Live Births
2006	25,972	13,270	12,702	15,148	19,041	41,120	4,265,593
2005	25,894	13,327	12,567	15,013	18,782	40,907	4,138,573
2004	26,001	13,068	12,933	14,836	18,602	40,837	4,112,055
2003	26,004	13,348	12,656	15,152	18,935	41,156	4,090,007

| | FETAL DEATHS | | | INFANT DEATHS | | | |
Year	Total*	20-27 Weeks	28 Weeks or More	Less Than 7 Days	Less Than 28 Days	Peri-natal Deaths	Live Births
2002	25,943	13,072	12,871	15,020	18,791	40,963	4,021,825
2001	26,373	13,122	13,251	14,622	18,275	40,995	4,026,036
2000	27,003	13,497	13,506	14,893	18,733	41,896	4,058,882
1999	26,884	13,457	13,427	14,874	18,700	41,758	3,959,417
1998	26,702	13,229	13,473	15,061	18,915	41,763	3,941,553
1997	26,486	12,800	13,686	14,827	18,507	41,313	3,880,894
1996	27,069	12,990	14,079	14,947	18,556	42,016	3,891,494
1995	27,294	13,043	14,251	15,483	19,186	42,777	3,899,589
1990	31,386	13,427	17,959	19,439	23,591	50,825	4,158,445
1985	29,661	10,958	18,703	21,317	25,573	50,978	3,760,833

*Fetal deaths with stated or presumed period of gestation of 20 weeks or more.
Modified from National Vital Statistics Reports, 60(8), August 28, 2012.
Source: CDC/NCHS, National Vital Statistics System.

EXERCISE 6-3
Mortality Data

1. How are the early neonatal, neonatal, perinatal, and infant rates different?

2. What is in the denominator of the ITOP rate?

3. Maternal mortality rates are those pregnancy-related deaths compared to obstetric admissions or _____.

4. What are the ranges for fetal deaths?

5. What are synonyms for adjusted rates?

6. Two means of normalizing populations are _____ and _____.

7. Which method of adjusting is applied when you multiply the age groupings of the observed population by the mortality rate of the US?

8. Calculate the following rates using the data provided in the table. Round to two decimal places.

Population Statistics for ABC State, 2016

Total mid-interval population	32,000,000
Total deaths	90,000
Maternal deaths	75
Obstetric admissions	2,000,000
ITOP	27,000
Infant deaths <8 days	10,000
Infant deaths 8-28 days	20,000
Infant deaths 28-365 days	25,000

EXERCISE 6-3
Mortality Data—cont'd

Population Statistics for ABC State, 2016

Live births	1,800,000
Total population women 15-44	15,000,000
Teenage pregnancies	350,000
Teenage mid-interval population	1,500,000
Late fetal deaths	5000

a. Crude death rate
b. Early neonatal mortality rate
c. Perinatal mortality rate
d. ITOP rate
e. Maternal mortality rate
f. Infant death rate

MORBIDITY DATA

Public health statistics that measure the occurrence of diseases, disorders, and injuries are called morbidity statistics. They allow for the tracking and trending of these disorders and help policy makers measure the effectiveness of their initiatives to reduce the *incidence* of specific conditions.

Reportable diseases, such as tuberculosis, measles, and rabies, are forwarded from individual physicians to their local health departments that record and again forward the report to the state and then finally the CDC. The study of the occurrences, causes, and patterns of health conditions is called **epidemiology**. When you hear the terms "epidemic," "pandemic," and "endemic," they refer to the particular spread of an outbreak of disease. An *epidemic* is the spread of a disease beyond a defined population. Examples of epidemics are influenza, typhus, and smallpox. A *pandemic* is a spread that encompasses more than one country or continent (like the pandemic of influenza in 1918 or the polio pandemic in the 1950s) and an *endemic* is the unexpected occurrence of a disease within a defined population. Influenza, along with chickenpox, are examples of endemics that occur within the US population.

Morbidity statistics are usually presented in the format of *incidence* and *prevalence* rates. **Incidence** rates are the number of new cases in a population divided by the population at risk, whereas **prevalence** rates are the number of new and existing cases of the disease/disorder again divided by the population at risk. While the first (incidence) is a measure of the onset of a disease, the second (prevalence) measures the public health burden existing within a particular population.

Measuring disease and disorders at the level of large populations is important to public health. Whether it is the incidence rate of measles in the population (Fig. 6-5), a rabies outbreak, or a newly emerging disease like Ebola hemorrhagic fever, health care providers (and the public) need the information to make decisions about how to manage the particular disorder.

Epidemiology The study of the occurrences, causes, and patterns of health conditions.

Incidence rate The number of new cases of a disease/disorder divided by the population at risk times a constant of 100,000.

Prevalence rate The number of new and existing cases of a disease/disorder in a population divided by the population at risk times a constant of 100,000.

TAKE AWAY

Incidence rates measure the new cases, while prevalence rates measure the new and existing cases.

Calculating Incidence

$$\frac{\text{Reported new cases of a disease for period}}{\text{Mid - interval population}} \times 1000 \text{ or more}$$

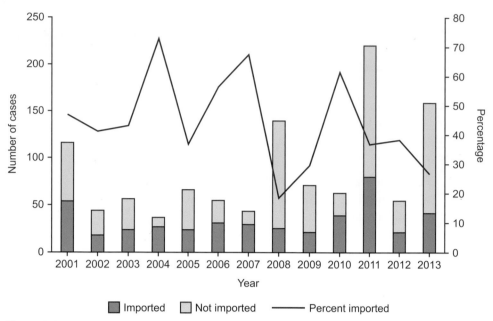

Figure 6-5 Number and percentage of measles cases that were directly imported and number of cases that were not directly imported[*]—United States, 2001 to 2013[†]. From: http://www.cdc.gov/mmwr/preview/mmwrhtml/mm6236a2.htm.

For example, say we wanted to calculate the incidence of concussions (or traumatic brain injuries, TBIs) among intercollegiate women's soccer players. In a given year, data show about 12,000 female athletes playing soccer at schools all over the country. During the same year, 541 TBIs are reported to the NCAA:

$$\frac{541}{12,000} \times 1000 = 45 \text{ concussions per } 1000 \text{ players}$$

Calculating Prevalence

$$\frac{\text{Reported new and existing cases of a disease for period}}{\text{Population during that time period}} \times 1000 \text{ or more}$$

Public health officials may want to know how widespread a disease is among certain groups, as a way of measuring its cost to the health care system. If there are 4,050,000 Americans living with generalized anxiety disorder (GAD) in 2015, and the population is estimated at 320 million, the prevalence would be

$$\frac{4,050,000}{320 \text{ million}} \times 1000 = 13 \text{ cases per } 1000 \text{ people}$$

However, physicians may diagnose 3 of the 4 million cases of GAD among women ages 25 and older, of whom there are 115 million in the country. What is the prevalence of GAD in that demographic?

---

[*]Directly imported cases are those in patients who acquired measles outside the United States and brought their infection into the United States. Cases not directly imported include those that were acquired in the United States but linked to directly imported cases, imported virus, and cases with unknown sources.
[†]As of Aug 24, 2013.

$$\frac{3\ \text{million}}{115\ \text{million}} \times 1000 = 26\ \text{cases per 1000 women ages 25 and older}$$

Because we narrowed the population to a specific demographic, we can see that GAD is twice as prevalent among adult women as it is among the rest of the population.

BRIEF CASE

FINDING MORBIDITY

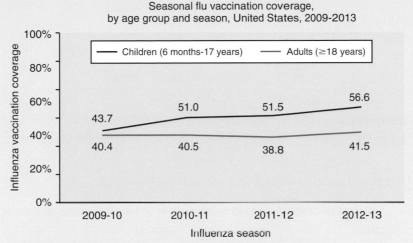

Seasonal flu vaccination coverage, by age group and season, United States, 2009-2013

Error bars represent 95% confidence intervals around the estimates.
The 2009-10 estimates do not include the influenza A (H1N1) pdm09 monovalent vaccine. Adult estimates for the 2011-12 and 2012-13 seasons reflect changes in methods of the Behavioral Risk Factor Surveillance System (BRFSS) (addition of cellular telephone sample and new weighting methods).

Before going to college, Michael had seen the advertisements for vaccines for flu, shingles, and meningitis. Now his infectious disease service is working with the oncology department to come up with statistics to help convince the administration of the need for more money for a compelling campaign to reach their community for the HPV vaccine. They are especially interested in their M/F ratios compared to the national stats to see if they should consider their targeted outreach differently than they are now. The national stats are readily available from the CDC for STIs that show 20 million new cases per year with a total of 110 million, along with figures for the total cost of treating them: $16 billion! HPV represents almost half of those cases, and it affects both sexes.

He picked up the estimated new cancer cases and deaths from the American Cancer Society 2015 Cancer Facts and Figures for cervical cancer (13,560 total with 3640 expected deaths).[4]

Next, he checked on the reported statistics for HPV-related cancers and found the following explanation of what HPV-attributable cancers are and how statistics can be used to determine the number of cancers most likely caused by HPV. For now, his request was just for a comparison of the cancer sites, although he thought his requestors might be interested in the entire table.

An HPV-attributable cancer is a cancer that is probably caused by HPV. HPV causes nearly all cervical cancers and many cancers of the anus, penis, vagina, vulva, and oropharynx. CDC studies used population-based data from cancer tissue to estimate the percentage of these cancers that are probably caused by HPV.

To find the number of HPV-attributable cancers, multiply the number of HPV-associated cancers by the percentage of these cancers that are probably caused by HPV. For example, about 4370 people are diagnosed with anal cancer each year, and about 91% of anal cancers are thought to be caused by HPV. 91% of 4370 is 3977, or about 4000, as shown in the table below.

Continued

BRIEF CASE—cont'd

	AVERAGE NUMBER OF CANCERS PER YEAR IN SITES WHERE HPV IS OFTEN FOUND (HPV-ASSOCIATED CANCERS)				NUMBER PROBABLY CAUSED BY HPV*		
Cancer Site	Male	Female	Both Sexes	Percentage Probably Caused by HPV	Male	Female	Both Sexes
Anus	1549 (1549/4370=35%)	2821 (2821/4370=65%)	4370	91%	1400	2600	4000
Cervix	0	11,422	11,422	91%	0	10,400	10,400
Oropharynx	9974 (9974/12417=80%)	2443 (2443/12417=20%)	12,417	72%	7200	1800	9000
Penis	1048	0	1048	63%	700	0	700
Vagina	0	735	735	75%	0	600	600
Vulva	0	3168	3168	69%	0	2200	2200
TOTAL	12,571	20,589	33,160		9,300	17,600	26,900

*Individual cells may not sum to total due to rounding.
Data are from all states meeting USCS publication criteria for all years 2006 to 2010 and cover approximately 94.8% of the US population.
From: Human Papillomavirus (HPV)-associated cancers. Centers for Disease Control and Prevention. Web page: http://www.cdc.gov/cancer/hpv/statistics/cases.htm.

Querying his own hospital system's data warehouse, Michael finds the following:

AVERAGE NUMBER OF CANCERS PER YEAR IN SITES WHERE HPV IS OFTEN FOUND (HPV-ASSOCIATED CANCERS)					
CANCER SITE	MALE	%	FEMALE	%	BOTH SEXES
Anus	106		365		
Cervix	0		569		
Oropharynx	277		31		
Penis	41		0		
Vagina	0		56		
Vulva	0		452		
Total					

Calculate the statistics for Michael's hospital and compare them to the national stats available. What is the male-to-female ratio for each type of cancer? How does his hospital compare in regard to the distribution of oropharyngeal and anal cancers by sex? What other analysis would you suggest that he perform to make his report more relevant?
[4]http://www.cancer.org/research/cancerfactsstatistics/cancerfactsfigures2015/index.

REVIEW QUESTIONS

1. How are public health and vital statistics different?

2. A confounding variable is one that can mask a trend. True or false?

3. Morbidity statistics measure disease. True or false?

4. The National Vital Statistics System is under the National Center for Healthcare _____ (Statistics).

5. The crude birth rate compares _____ to _____.

6. Why are adjusted rates helpful in comparing two populations?

7. Both methods of adjustment use population proportions and _____ rates.

8. Which method of adjusting is applied when you multiply the mortality rate of the population you are examining by the US proportion?

9. Indirect adjustment gives you an expected number of deaths, while the direct adjustment calculation gives you an expected _____ rate.

10. The standardized mortality ratio (SMR) compares the total number of deaths in the population to the _____ number of deaths in the population.

11. Using the following tables, calculate expected mortality rates for California for each of the age ranges and the state as a whole. Then, using the direct method, calculate the adjusted mortality rate for California using the appropriate population proportions.

CALIFORNIA

Age Range	Deaths	Population	Crude Death Rate	Pop Prop
0-9	3100	5,037,172	61.5424687	0.13521173
10-19	1449	5,414,870	26.7596452	0.1453502
20-44	12,551	13,266,536	94.6064594	0.3561108
45-64	46,708	9,288,864	502.838668	0.249339
65+	170,176	4,246,514	4007.42821	0.11398827
Total	233,984	37,253,956	628.078264	

United States

Age Range	Deaths	Population	Crude Death Rate	Pop Prop
0-9	31,232	40,550,019	77.0209257	0.13133799
10-19	13,836	42,717,537	32.3895079	0.13835839
20-44	130,956	103,720,553	126.258486	0.33594187
45-64	494,009	81,489,445	606.224524	0.26393724
65+	1,798,276	40,267,984	4465.77112	0.13042451
	2,468,309	308,745,538	799.463861	1

12. The population of women from 15 to 44 is used in which rates?

13. A late fetal death is after _____ weeks.

14. The _____ rate compares new cases of a disorder to the population at risk.

15. Neonatal deaths are those under the first _____ days of life.

16. Teen pregnancy rates compare births in the population of women from ages _____ to 19.

17. Early fetal deaths are those that occur before _____ weeks.

18. Late fetal deaths are included in the denominator of the _____ death rate.

19. The numerator of ITOP rates is _____.

20. Natality refers to _____.

21. Given the following tabled data, calculate the rates. Round all figures to a whole number.

Measure	Total
Population	3,170,000
Deaths	4293
Infant deaths <8 days	51
Deaths <28 days	76
Late fetal deaths	34
Live births	4791
Tuberculosis, new cases	25
Tuberculosis, existing cases	110 cases
Mortality 15-24 for TB	3
Population 15-24	250,334

a. crude mortality rate:
b. specific mortality rate of age set 15 to 24 for TB:
c. neonatal mortality rate:
d. TB prevalence rate:
e. incidence rate:

CHAPTER 7

DEPARTMENTAL DATA

CHAPTER OUTLINE

MEASURES OF PRODUCTIVITY
    Transcription
    Coding

Document Imaging
Release of Information
REIMBURSEMENT STATISTICS

Prospective Payment System
Case Mix Index
COMPLIANCE STATISTICS
REVIEW QUESTIONS

KEY TERMS

base rate
case mix index (CMI)
delinquent record count

diagnosis-related group (DRG)
productivity standard
prospective payment system (PPS)

push rate
relative weight (RW)
rolling quarterly average

LEARNING OBJECTIVES

At the end of the chapter, you should be able to:

1. Apply productivity standards to various functions within HIM.
2. Demonstrate understanding of inpatient prospective payment systems (DRG) and case mix index, and how the calculations are performed.
3. Examine case mix index data to identify trends.
4. Analyze case mix index data to identify fraudulent coding trends.
5. Understand delinquency rate calculations for accreditation purposes.

A variety of statistics are calculated within the HIM department to assist in planning, staffing, and controlling departmental functions. Although not every facility computes all of these various numbers, HIM professionals should be aware of what these statistics mean and their value to management and decision-making.

BRIEF CASE

MANAGING THE DEPARTMENT

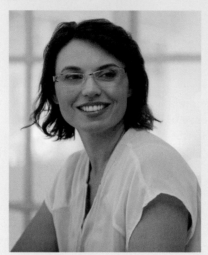

Ana, the HIM assistant director, has been asked by her supervisor, Janet, to begin collecting data for the upcoming facility budget discussions. Ana knows that she must refresh her Excel spreadsheet skills for salary tabulations and other calculations used in the budgeting and management of the facility. Ana is also responsible for employee evaluations, and she knows that objective productivity measurements are important to fairly evaluate team members in all job functions. Data analysis is Ana's favorite part of the job and every year at budget planning time, she feels that her role, and the data produced in HIM, becomes much more visible and important to the entire facility.

MEASURES OF PRODUCTIVITY

Within the HIM department, managers track how much work is being done to determine how much staffing is needed, the performance of the current staff, and the cost incurred by various HIM department activities. How many charts can we abstract in a day or in an hour? How long does it take to scan 1000 pages of paper into the EHR? Productivity is the unit of performance defined by management in quantitative standards, measuring *how much* is being done.

Generally, the goal of a manager is to keep the amount of work both even and meaningful. Periods of frenzied work create the opportunity for errors and are hard on employees, while downtime is a waste of staff skills and, in the end, a waste of money. To avoid these situations, **productivity standards** are in place to keep the pace of the workflow smooth. For example, if productivity standards dictate that an outpatient surgery coder is required to code seven records per hour, and at this facility the physicians typically perform 100 to 120 procedures per day, you can anticipate that two full-time outpatient coders working eight-hour days will be able to complete all the coding each day (see Box 7-1).

You might be wondering how we know that coding seven records per hour is an appropriate rate. Perhaps this is too slow, and an efficient coder could process nine records of this size per hour? To find out, HIM managers can look for benchmarks in the industry—the productivity levels of other facilities. Asking other HIM department directors in the same city or region is also a valuable way to check productivity levels because this limits geographical differences to provide a consistent measure. However, employee responsibilities can vary from facility to facility, so knowing the unique tasks performed by individuals in the department is important for accuracy.

● **Productivity standard** An expectation of the amount of work performed.

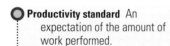

7 records per hour × 8 hours per day = 56 records per coder per day. 56 × 2 coders = 112 records. What if each coder could only code 5 records an hour, but there only 75 procedures per day? 5 × 8 = 40, and 75 ÷ 40 = 1.875, so two full-time coders would still be optimal.

> **BOX 7-1**
>
> **FULL-TIME EQUIVALENTS (FTES)**
> . . . .
>
> When considering productivity, productive time is considered to be 8 hours of an 8.5 hour day. Full-time employees (FTE) are usually considered to be working a 40 hour work week, 52 weeks a year (260 days), with a total of 2080 hours in a year. Employers pay more for employees than just their wages; however, vacation time and other paid time off, retirement contributions, along with a portion of health insurance and taxes such as Social Security and Medicare, must all be calculated as part of the cost of an employee. Such benefits are often calculated at 30% more than the employee's wages.

In all aspects of HIM, including coding, release of information, and document imaging, the amount of work varies depending on whether the care provided is inpatient, outpatient, or emergency department. Timing each employee on these various work types will provide you with baseline standards that can be derived from an average of the particular work type in question. Many HIM departments set a goal just slightly above the average, called a **push rate**. For example, in an outpatient setting, the fastest coder might code 10 records per hour, while the slowest codes five. A standard could be set at seven, but if you want to challenge your employees, you could set a push rate of eight or nine records per hour.

> ● **Push rate** A productivity standard slightly higher than the average or usual amount of work completed.

Other duties must also be calculated in, which will differ depending on the functions performed at each unique working environment. For example, answering the phone can be very time-consuming, and it might be most fair to rotate the responsibility so everyone has a day for this. For coders, writing queries or searching for transcribed documents may take extra time. In the document imaging area, employees who prepare medical records for scanning (preppers) will need time to remove staples, tape any torn sheets, and flatten any folded sheets prior to feeding stacks of records through the scanner. Release of information employees need to carefully review the consent form, but if a nonstandard form is submitted such as a handwritten note or even a typed letter, then the review will be slowed down. In the following pages, we will explore the factors involved in calculating productivity levels for the common positions in the HIM department.

> **TAKE AWAY** ●· · · · · · · · ·
>
> Performance standards can be used to judge whether employees are meeting expectations and to encourage employees to improve their performance.

Transcription

The rate of transcription, the conversion of digital auditory files to text, has been measured for many years. Medical transcriptionists (Figure 7-1) may be paid by the hour, by production of lines, or by a combination of the two with bonus incentive pay for production above the established standard. The counting of lines and what constitutes a line vary by facility and will not be examined in depth here, but typically 65 characters = one line. As voice recognition technology has advanced and become commonplace, transcriptionists' job duties have shifted from primarily typing to an editing function. Examples of transcription production will be used to better understand the standards and how workflow can be impacted. This area of HIM has standards in place that are comparable across most work settings.

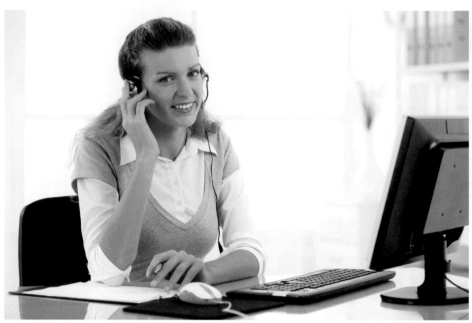

Figure 7-1 A medical transcriptionist entering lines of dictation.

✎ Calculating Productivity Based on Completed Work

$$\text{Productivity} = \frac{\text{Completed Work}}{\text{Time Period}}$$

Recall that an FTE working 40-hour weeks, 52 weeks a year, at 8 hours a day will work 260 days in a year, not taking sick, holiday, or vacation days into account. So let us say Darrell, a transcriptionist who has been with the department for 1 year, produced 286,000 lines last year. To calculate his daily production, we would divide 286,000 lines by the days worked, which is 260.

$$\text{Productivity} = \frac{286,000 \text{ lines}}{260 \text{ days}} = 1100 \text{ lines per day for the year}$$

Darrell's average productivity is 1100 lines per day. Most employees, however, do not work a full 260 days in a year—they take time off for vacations, holidays, and sick days. Darrell's coworker, Kyleigh, produced about the same number of lines last year (285,000), but she had two weeks of vacation (10 days), had three holidays off, and called off sick four times. Subtracting these 17 days from 260, our equation is:

$$\text{Productivity} = \frac{285,000}{260 - 17} = 1172.84 \text{ lines per day}$$

Because Kyleigh is a little more productive than Darrell, she output about the same amount of work in less time.

Calculating Unit Cost

Once we know how many lines a transcriptionist can produce in a day, a month, or in an hour, we can use that employee's wages or salary to determine how much it costs to pay that person for each line produced. The formula for calculating unit cost for a year is below.

$$\text{Unit Cost} = \frac{\text{Annual Compensation}}{\text{Annual Productivity}}$$

In this case, the unit is each line transcribed. To continue our example, let us say Darrell earns $14.00 per hour. Converting this to annual compensation, Darrell worked 2080 hours in a year × $14.00 per hour = $29,120 per year. If you add 30% for benefits (see Box 7-1):

Darrell earns $29,120 per year × 1.3 benefits cost = $37,856 per year

The total cost to pay Darrell is $37,856 each year. Plugging this figure along with his total annual productivity into our formula, we get

$$\text{Unit Cost} = \frac{\$37,856}{286,000 \text{ lines}} = \$0.1324, \text{ or about 13.2 cents per line}$$

Let us look at another example, Ananya, a transcriptionist whose average output is 1600 lines per day—significantly higher than Darrell. Because of her vacation and other earned time off, she worked 240 days this year.

1600 lines × 240 days = 384,000 lines

Ananya may have only worked 1920 hours this year after her vacations and other paid time off (240 days × 8 hours = 1920), but she is much more efficient. Even at her higher pay of $18.00 per hour, we calculate her unit cost as follows:

$18.00 per hour × 2080 hours paid per year = $37,440 per year

Adding in 30% for the cost of Ananya's employee benefits:

$37,440 × 1.3 = $48,672

So, to calculate Ananya's unit cost:

$$\text{Unit Cost} = \frac{\$48,672}{384,000 \text{ lines}} = \$0.12675, \text{ or about 12.7 cents per line}$$

Even though Ananya was at work 20 days fewer than Darrell, and we paid her for it, because she is more productive, she is cheaper per unit. This example points out that a more productive employee will result in a lower cost per unit. Labor cost is less for a more productive employee.

When overflow levels of transcription are faced, such as during peak census times or if a transcriptionist is out for an extended time, it may be necessary to outsource dictation to keep the workflow moving. Transcription vendors charge by the line, which is

TAKE AWAY ●·········

The per unit cost for a more productive employee will be lower than that of a less productive employee why it is useful to know what your transcription staff unit cost is. Vendors may charge 15 cents a line or more depending on the required turnaround time, work type, medical staff makeup, etc.

Calculating Staff Levels Based on Volume

$$\text{FTEs} = \frac{\text{Volume of Dictation}}{\text{Productivity}}$$

Using the volume of dictation and staff productivity, an HIM manager can determine the number of employees needed. Let us say our average transcriptionist types 125 lines per hour (1000 lines per 8 hour productive work day × 5 work days = 5000 lines per week). This would result in 20,000 lines typed per month, or 60,000 lines typed for a 3 month period. If over the 3 months of March, April, and May last year (92 days including weekends) your facility physicians created 183,315 lines of dictation, the calculation for the number of FTEs looks as follows:

$$\text{FTEs} = \frac{183,315}{60,000} = 3.06 \text{ FTEs}$$

We need three full-time transcriptionists to cover the anticipated volume of work.

BRIEF CASE

ERASING THE BACKLOG

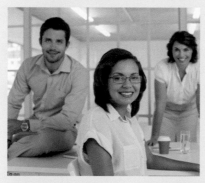

Ana is tasked with the job of figuring out how to catch up a recent transcription backlog and needs to do some calculations on productivity and cost. Her lead transcriptionist had gone out on medical leave unexpectedly, and despite constant contacts with her temporary agency, there were no replacements in sight. While the lead transcriptionist, Maria, would be back in 2 weeks, the backlog remained and would continue to grow until her return. The total backlog is projected to be 17,500 lines. One off-site agency proposed a rate of $0.21/line and a turnaround of 2 weeks for a total cost of $3675.

After consulting with her director, Ana proposed an incentive program to erase the backlog with the department's other four transcriptionists. She created an incentive pay of time and a half; this amounts to $0.18/line for the top two transcriptionists ($0.12 × 1.5 = $0.18) and $0.12/line for the less productive transcriptionists ($0.08 × 1.5 = $0.12 per line). She assumes the work will be split equally among the four transcriptionists on staff. Using the data presented in the chart below, how long will it take and how much will it cost to erase the backlog? For length of time, you need to state the range of days to completion among the transcriptionists. How does Ana's proposal compare with the outside agency?

BRIEF CASE—cont'd

ERASING THE BACKLOG

TRANS.	AVG LINES/ DAY	EXTRA LINES FOR INCENTIVE PAY	COST/ LINE FOR NORMAL TIME	PROJECTED INCENTIVE PAY/LINE FOR ADDITIONAL WORK	DAYS TO COMPLETE ADDITIONAL LINES	COST/ TRANSCRIPTIONIST FOR EXTRA LINES (BACKLOG)
Aisha	1270	4375	0.12	0.18		
Brianna	730	4375	0.08	0.12		
Charles	850	4375	0.08	0.12		
Darlene	1150	4375	0.12	0.18		
Total	4000	17,500	X	X		

Coding

For coding, different productivity levels are necessary for inpatient, outpatient, and emergency department (ED) records because each requires a different level of patient care. Think about how much more information is contained in an inpatient record than an outpatient surgery record. It is reasonable to expect inpatient coding productivity standards in the three to five records per hour range, whereas outpatient (ambulatory) surgery standards may be seven to nine records per hour. ED records tend to be the least complex and shortest, so coding productivity standards may be 18 to 20 records per hour.

As with transcriptionists, we can use productivity to determine the number of coding FTEs we need in the department. Let us say that your standard and average speed for outpatient records is 19 ED charts per hour. Your emergency room saw 6000 patients in March. If you have two full-time coders and one half-time coder assigned to this task, can they keep up with the workflow?

Let us start by determining how many ED charts the three coders can code in a day. First, we add up the number of hours worked by all three coders in a working day. The full-time employees each work 8 hours, and the half-time coder works 4 hours:

$$8 \text{ hours} + 8 \text{ hours} + 4 \text{ hours} = 20 \text{ hours}$$

Then, multiply by 19, the number of charts each can code in an hour:

$$19 \text{ charts} \times 20 \text{ hours in a day} = 380 \text{ ED charts per day}$$

On a given day, the coding staff should be able to code 380 ED records based on the productivity standard. Lastly, we need to determine how many productive days there are in March, but before you flip back to the knuckle counting song we learned in Chapter 2, be careful! We need to count how many days the HIM department is open and the coders are working, not the total days in the month. In a month with 20 productive work days:

$$380 \text{ ED charts} \times 20 \text{ days} = 7600 \text{ charts per month}$$

With three coders at this volume, it looks like the ED coders are overstaffed. They are capable of coding 7600 charts per month, while the facility only generated 6000 records. An HIM department manager in this position might consider letting the part-time coder go, cutting hours of the full-time coders, or training one of these ED coders in a more difficult type of coding (outpatient surgery or inpatient) depending on the facility's needs.

ED Emergency department.

TAKE AWAY •·········

The time it takes to perform many HIM functions depends on the complexity of the medical record.

FTE Full-time equivalent.

Document Imaging

In many facilities, patient care is recorded on paper at the point-of-care (POC), and these pages are later scanned into the electronic health record (EHR) as images (Figure 7-2). A full discussion of imaging and the different types of EHR systems is beyond the scope of this text, but Table 7-1 lists the several functions performed by the HIM department during document imaging.

Document imaging productivity can be measured by the volume of images handled—the number of pieces of paper to be digitized—or by the inches or weight of the paper. As noted earlier, types of records scanned (emergency department, outpatient, inpatient) should also be factored into the standards since each type of care represents a different level of complexity.

Let us do some practice calculations to figure how much time and staff are needed to process a given workload. Looking at a sample stack of files, you estimate that each folder is about 3/4s of an inch think and therefore contains about 150 pages. If we had 1802 discharges in March, how many employees are required for the functions above?

EHR Electronic health record.

○ MATH REVIEW

For the purpose of estimating workload, it might be necessary to calculate the number of images in a given file thickness. If there are 200 pieces of paper in an inch (stacked) and your average chart thickness is three-quarters of an inch, how many pieces of paper would this equal? 0.75 inches×200=150 pieces of paper per record, on average, at your facility. We are assuming that all pages of the record are printed on one side only with this example, and therefore, our pages per record is equal to our images.

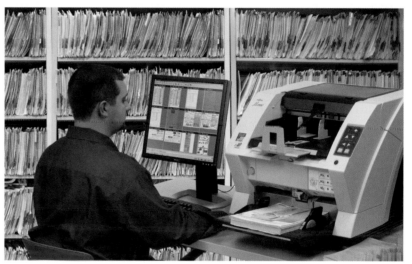

Figure 7-2 An HIM department staffer scans paper portions of the patient's medical record into the EHR. (Courtesy Fujitsu Computer Products of America, Inc.)

TABLE 7-1	
DOCUMENT IMAGING TASKS	
TASK	**DESCRIPTION**
Document preparation	Ensures the pages of the record will feed properly into the scanner; removes staples, checks for tears, assembles record properly
Scanning	Ensures the records are properly fed into the scanner
Quality control	Views digitized images of the records on the screen to ensure pages are scanned properly
Indexing	Ensures the digitized record is searchable by patient name, date of birth, and medical record number

First, let us use some historical averages for a given facility to estimate how many pages (or images) of a record can be processed each hour for each task in the document imaging process. Based on the past productivity in a given HIM department, the supervisor expects rates as follows:

Document Preparation: 400 pages/hr
Scanning: 1800 pages/hr
Quality Control: 1800 pages/hr
Indexing: 750 pages/hr

Next, we will determine the number of images we have total for the month.

$$1802 \text{ discharges} \times 150 \text{ images} = 270,300 \text{ images in March}$$

Third, we can take the total number of images we estimate for March (270,300) and divide it by the average baseline we expect to process each hour.

$$\frac{270,300 \text{ images}}{400 \text{ prepped per hour}} = 675.75 \text{ hours to prep all the images.}$$

That is too much work for one person, of course. An FTE usually works 40 hours a week, or 160 hours a month (40 hours × 4 weeks). So the final calculation divides the total work hours for the task by the number of hours one FTE works in a month.

$$\frac{675.75 \text{ hours}}{160 \text{ hours}} = 4.22 \text{ full-time equivalent employees}$$

The calculations show that just for the prepping, the department needs about four people working full time (or three full-time and two part-time employees, or many other combinations). The math for the remaining document imaging tasks looks as follows:

Task	Average Productivity or Performance Standard	Total Images (Discharges × Images per Record)	Work Hours (Total Images ÷ Standard)	FTEs Needed (Work Hours ÷ 160 Hours per Month)
Document preparation	400	$1802 \times 150 = 270,300$	$\frac{270,300}{400} = 675.75 \text{ hours}$	$\frac{675.75}{160} = 4.22 \text{ FTEs}$
Scanning	1800		$\frac{270,300}{1800} = 150.17 \text{ hours}$	$\frac{150.17}{160} = 0.94 \text{ FTEs}$
Quality control	1800		$\frac{270,300}{1800} = 150.17 \text{ hours}$	$\frac{150.17}{160} = 0.94 \text{ FTEs}$
Indexing	750		$\frac{270,300}{750} = 360.40 \text{ hours}$	$\frac{360.40}{160} = 2.25 \text{ FTEs}$

Therefore, we would need just over 8 FTEs to keep the workflow current in document imaging for March. Cross-training employees in the various functions of prepping, scanning, quality control, and indexing would allow you to spread the work out evenly and also would help account for any absences. Also, recall that we used the historical average to calculate each function. There could be room to use a push rate to increase productivity.

● **ROI** Release of information.

Release of Information

Release of information (ROI) is an HIM function that includes the tracking of requests for documentation within the health record, checking the validity of the request, retrieving the specified information from the record, and sending it to the requestor. Requestors include physicians, patients, insurance companies, workman's compensation, disability, risk management, and lawyers. With the advent of the HITECH Act, part of the American Recovery and Reinvestment Act (ARRA) of 2009, a new set of requestors, federal auditors, began to compose a major portion of the volume of requests. These auditors use information in the medical record to determine if overpayment or improper billing has occurred. Federal auditors including Recovery Audit Contractors (RACs), Medicare Administrative Contractors (MACs), Medicaid Integrity Contractors (MICs), Zone Program Integrity Contractors (ZPICs), and Comprehensive Error Rate Testing (CERTs) have greatly increased the number of pages requested.

While paper records were previously mailed, scanned, or faxed, electronic records can now be encrypted for sending, and tracked digitally. The ROI staffer often uses software to assist in ROI tasks, including
- the logging and tracking of requests
- verification of the patient's identity
- determining the required turnaround time
- retrieving the information requested
- verifying the authorization
- sending the information
- billing for the service

Managing ROI includes not only complying with the requirements for legal disclosure but also calculating the staff and costs required to complete the requests. The number of staff required for the position will depend on the number of requests received. A hypothetical hospital has 31,000 pages of requests per year that are managed by one FTE. If the number of requests doubled to 60,000 per year, the director would be able to justify two individuals to handle the workload.

 Calculating ROI Costs

The cost of requests can be calculated as the salary of the ROI position divided by the number of pages or requests handled per year.

$$\frac{\text{Salary of ROI staff}}{\text{Number of pages or number of requests} \times \text{day worked}}$$

For example, an ROI staffer might average 130 pages per day and his/her salary, including benefits, is $32,000. After 10 vacation days, 5 holidays, and 5 sick days, he/she works 240 days in a year. To plug those values into our formula:

$$\frac{\$32,000}{130 \text{ pages} \times 240 \text{ working days}} = \frac{\$32,000}{31,200 \text{ pages per year}} = \$1.03 \text{ per page}$$

EXERCISE 7-1

Measure of Productivity

1. The physicians at the group practice usually need 65,000 lines of dictation transcribed each month. If the minimum productivity standard is 110 lines per hour, and there are 20 working days in a month, how many FTEs does the practice need to employ?

2. Flip makes $17.50 per hour as an inpatient coder. He works 35 hours a week and gets two weeks of paid vacation a year. If he codes an average of 3.5 charts per hour, how many charts can he code in a year? How much does it cost for Flip to code each chart?

EXERCISE 7-1

Measure of Productivity—cont'd

3. A physician clinic sees 350 patients per day. Using the emergency room coder productivity standard of 19 charts per hour, with a 6-hour productive work day, how many coders would the clinic need to hire?

4. In a given month, the emergency room coders logged the following:

   Coder A: 2800 ER charts coded, worked 8 hours per day, 20 days
   Coder B: 2100 ER charts coded, worked 8 hours per day, 20 days
   Coder C: 1100 ER charts coded, worked 4 hours per day, 20 days

   How many minutes is it currently taking each coder to code one ER record?
   HINT: You will need to calculate the number of minutes worked in the time
   period. Who is the least productive coder?

5. A small hospital has an average of 55 requests per week with an average of 4 pages each. The salary of the position for handling the requests is $29,000. What is the cost per page of answering a request?

REIMBURSEMENT STATISTICS

In Chapter 4, we saw how the bed count, ALOS, occupancy percentage, and other measures can tell us how much of a hospital's resources—its staff and space within the facility—is being used. But besides space and staffing concerns, all providers, regardless of whether they are for-profit or not-for-profit, state-run, or private, need to know about the cost of providing health care. How much does it cost to treat our patients? What types of cases do we usually treat? How much money can we expect to receive from the patient's third-party payer?

Medicare, administered by the Centers for Medicare and Medicaid (CMS), is the largest payer in the United States, though many individuals have health insurance coverage through their employer and private insurers, such as Blue Cross/Blue Shield. These payers determine payment to providers not on the basis of individual services, but by aggregating data to see how much it costs to treat certain diagnoses and/or provide certain procedures.

Prospective Payment System

Using a **prospective payment system (PPS),** Medicare and other payers calculate that certain diagnoses and/or procedures **use the same amount of resources**. Therefore, the amount paid to the provider (the reimbursement) is the same for all patients whose care falls under a given group of diagnoses. These groups or categories, containing similar diagnoses for inpatient stays, where patients require use of similar resources, are called **diagnosis-related groups (DRGs)**.

Stat Tip

CMS calls their DRG system MS-DRGs, where the "MS" stands for Medicare Severity. Some other payers use the AP-DRG system, where "AP" stands for "all-payer," and "APR-DRG," where the R is for refined and includes medical severity.

Prospective payment system (PPS) A system used by payers, primarily the Centers for Medicare and Medicaid Services (CMS), for reimbursing acute care facilities on the basis of statistical analysis of health care data.

Diagnosis-related groups (DRGs) A collection of health care descriptions organized into statistically similar categories.

CMS Centers for medicare and medicaid services.

PPS Prospective payment system.

CC Complications or comorbidities.

MCC Major complications or comorbidities.

TAKE AWAY

The DRGs used in a prospective payment system help us anticipate the cost of providing care and the monetary reimbursement expected.

ALOS Average length of stay.

Relative weight (RW) A number assigned yearly by the Centers for Medicare and Medicaid Services (CMS) that is applied to each diagnosis-related group (DRG) and used to calculate reimbursement. This number represents the comparative difference in the use of resources by patients in each DRG.

Case mix index The arithmetic average (mean) of the relative diagnosis-related group weights of all health care cases in a given period.

Base rate A standardized dollar amount used with an individual DRG to determine payment.

For example, the payer may look at thousands of patients who have undergone a procedure to implant a permanent pacemaker for a heart condition. Costs associated with this procedure would include the housekeeping services and staffing while the patient is in the hospital, fees to the surgeon, the cost of the device and other surgical supplies, and nursing care before, during, and after the procedure. Examining these data, they find that historically patients who undergo this procedure and who have no complications from the surgery stay in the hospital an average of 3 days, with average total costs of $20,000. Medicare and other payers using PPS then determine their reimbursement based on these averages and pay providers $20,000 for *all* patients who undergo this treatment at this facility, regardless of the actual cost to treat an individual patient. This type of patient is grouped into DRG 244, "Permanent cardiac pacemaker implant W/O CC/MCC"—meaning that the implant was *without complications or comorbidities* (CC) *or major complications or comorbidities* (MCC). If a patient stays 2 or 4 days instead of 3, the hospital still receives $20,000; the same is true if the patient uses less resources. By classifying patients into DRGs, health care providers and third-party payers can predict the amount of resources used and the reimbursement expected for each DRG.

Let us look at another example: patients who are admitted to the hospital with severe migraine headaches. These patients are grouped into DRG 103, "Headaches W/O MCC," and we also expect an ALOS of 3 days. They may stay in the facility for the same length of time as the patients who had a pacemaker implanted (an average of 3 days), but the patients with migraines used far fewer resources. These patients did not require use of the operating room, for example, and did not need the postoperative care provided after surgery. The patients in DRG 103 have a lower *relative weight (RW)* than our pacemaker patients in DRG 244.

Each DRG is assigned a **relative weight (RW)** by CMS, such that a weight of 2 is twice as resource intensive as a weight of 1, and a weight of 0.5 uses half as many resources as a relative weight of 1. In other words, the relative weight of 2 would indicate that the diagnosis is more complex, and the patient would consume twice as many resources for treatment of the condition. According to Medicare's 2014 MS-DRG figures, our patient hospitalized for headaches (DRG 103) has a relative weight of 1.0430, while the pacemaker implant patient requires more than twice the amount of resources, with a relative weight of 2.1608. The DRG relative weights are adjusted by CMS annually on October 1st.

DRGs and their RWs provide the basis for determining monetary reimbursement amounts to health care providers, but the actual amount of reimbursement depends on several factors. CMS considers the average wage in the area, and where the facility is located (geographically). Location can be urban, rural, or a sole community provider of a specific service. It also considers the type of institution, such as teaching versus nonteaching, and the volume of low-income patients. In addition, when determining reimbursement, CMS and other payers consider the **case mix index (CMI)**, the mean of the DRG weights for a health care provider over a certain period of time. Because of factors like these, each facility is assigned a unique **base rate**, which is also adjusted annually on October 1st. The base rate is the standardized dollar amount that the facility will then use to multiply by the relative weight of each DRG to determine payment.

Calculating Base Rate for a DRG

$$\text{Payment} = \text{facility base rate} \times \text{DRG relative weight (RW)}$$

So, if the base rate for the facility is $1100.00 and the relative weight for a certain DRG is 2, then the payment for that DRG is $2200.00. The following table illustrates how different types of patients and the corresponding DRG relative weights impact payment to the facility.

Description	DRG	Relative Weight	Base Rate	Payment
Coronary artery disease with angioplasty and stent	248	2.9396	$2200	$6467.12
Coronary bypass with angioplasty	231	7.9084	$2200	$17,398.48
Cardiomyopathy with heart transplant	001	24.2794	$2200	$53,414.68

If you multiply the number of patients for each DRG, you can get an idea about the resource usage for your facility, and you can also analyze which DRG has generated the most revenue for your facility. The chief financial officer (CFO) is very interested in the types of patients (and the DRG assignments) that your hospital is treating because this influences revenue. This information is useful in determining what types of services to expand, the types of equipment to purchase, and which DRGs are losing money for the hospital.

In the example that follows, you can see that DRG C generates the most revenue even though the relative weight is higher for DRG A. Also, even though DRG B has more patients, the relative weight is lower, so the impact is less overall.

$$DRG\ A = 523\ patients \times 2.0330 = 1063.2590$$

$$DRG\ B = 689\ patients \times 0.9960 = 686.2440$$

$$DRG\ C = 602\ patients \times 1.9460 = 1171.4920$$

$$DRG\ D = 586\ patients \times 1.4530 = 851.4580$$

● CFO Chief financial officer.

Stat Tip

Note that with DRG and CMI calculation, you carry the answer to the decimal plus four digits, X.XXXX, to capture the details of these weights.

BRIEF CASE

IDENTIFYING REVENUE SOURCES

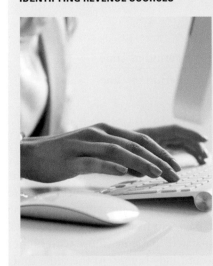

CMS adjusts relative weights annually, and Ana needs to present the new revenue projections to the CFO. Calculate the new relative weights based on the increases noted and then recalculate the impact on these DRGs treated at the facility. What changes do you see, and how do you interpret the changes?

BRIEF CASE—cont'd

IDENTIFYING REVENUE SOURCES

	INITIAL RELATIVE WEIGHT	RELATIVE WEIGHT CHANGE	NEW RELATIVE WEIGHT	NEW TOTAL WEIGHT	BASE RATE EXAMPLE (×$1100)
A = 523 patients	2.0330	15%			
B = 689 patients	0.9960	18%			
C = 602 patients	1.9460	4%			
D = 586 patients	1.4530	10%			

TAKE AWAY ●·········

The CMI number could be said to represent the average DRG weight, and therefore the complexity of the cases treated.

Case Mix Index

The case mix index is a measure of the relative cost needed to treat the mix of patients at a given facility. If you multiply this "average" by the base rate that is assigned to the facility, you can get an idea of what types of patients it treats and how many of your resources (how much money) those patients will consume. In addition, you can calculate how much money your facility can expect to receive for reimbursement for future budgetary projections.

Let us look at an example, using our initial DRG figures. After multiplying each DRG occurrence by the relative weight, all of those totals can be added up and divided by the number of patients to arrive at the case mix index for that facility.

DRG	**Patients LY**	**RW**	**Weight Total**
DRG A	523 patients	× 2.0330	= 1063.2590
DRG B	689 patients	× 0.9960	= 686.2440
DRG C	602 patients	× 1.9460	= 1171.4920
DRG D	586 patients	× 1.4530	= 851.4580
	2400 patients		**3772.4530**

To calculate the case mix index, we sum the weight totals and divide by the total number of patients.

 Calculating Case Mix Index

$$\text{Case Mix Index} = \frac{\text{Total Weights for a Period of Time}}{\text{Total Patients for a Period of Time}}$$

$$\frac{3772.4530}{2400} = 1.5718554$$

For these four DRGs, our case mix index is 1.5719.

This case mix index number could be said to represent the average DRG weight for our patients. We can convert that to relative cost by multiplying by our hospital's base rate. With the base rate of $1100.00 used earlier, for our 2400 patients represented in the example, we would expect to receive $4,149,816 in payment from Medicare ($1100 × 2400 × 1.5719 = $4,149,816). If we treat more "complicated" patients (those with higher DRG weights), then our reimbursement will be accordingly higher. At the same time,

remember that the total reimbursement is also dependent on the volume of patients—
so that one heart transplant patient with an extremely high weight will not bring in as
much revenue as a large number of patients with a much lower weight.

Remember, Medicare uses a prospective payment system, and this means that payment
is based on the diagnosis/DRG that best describes the patient's condition and treatment.
Based on average daily census showing the number of patients currently in the hospital,
the HIM department and the CFO can concurrently calculate the amount of money the
facility will receive for treating patients under Medicare and other payers using DRGs.
These revenues are important for a facility to know when the budgeting process begins.
Using DRGs and the case mix, a facility can project how much money it will have to
spend on equipment upgrades and other improvements in the years to come.

Although tracking trends in case mix is useful in predicting the financial viability of
an institution, it can also point to potentially fraudulent coding practices. Complications and comorbidities increase the weight of DRGs and lead to higher CMIs. When
the complications and comorbidities are not documented but are included in the grouping process, the hospital may be liable for fraud. Data mining at the national and local
level is able to trend CMIs for similar hospitals over time and determine if a hospital's
CMI is outside normal limits, which could suggest upcoding or other types of fraud.

BRIEF CASE

CASE MIX INVESTIGATION

The hospital CFO has requested the latest CMI calculations. Ana is well aware of the
revenue projections that the CFO will make based on the CMI report and that the
accuracy of the data is extremely important.

Ana calculates the facility case mix index and notices that it is higher than last year
and closer to the national average, shown below. A new cardiology physician group
joined the medical staff last year, and Ana knows the rise in case mix index can be at-
tributed to the more resource-intensive patients the facility is now treating.

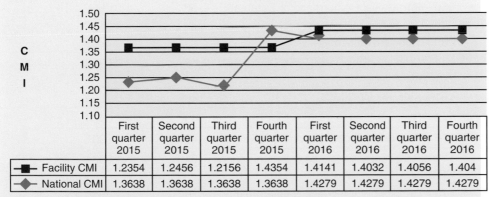

Comparison of facility CMI to National CMI 2015-2016

	First quarter 2015	Second quarter 2015	Third quarter 2015	Fourth quarter 2015	First quarter 2016	Second quarter 2016	Third quarter 2016	Fourth quarter 2016
■ Facility CMI	1.2354	1.2456	1.2156	1.4354	1.4141	1.4032	1.4056	1.404
◆ National CMI	1.3638	1.3638	1.3638	1.3638	1.4279	1.4279	1.4279	1.4279

Quarter

A closer analysis of the average CMI by coder revealed that there were sizable differences between average CMIs for the existing coders and the average facility CMI
beginning with the fourth quarter of 2015. What if the rise in the facility CMI was not
due to the more complex diagnoses of the cardiology practice. Could the uptick in the
CMI indicate a fraudulent practice, such as upcoding? What was not readily available
was the CMI average for the new coder, Frances, who came with the cardiology practice. Using the chart below, finish filling in the chart that Ana used to analyze the coding
department's CMI by coder.

BRIEF CASE—cont'd

CMI AVERAGES PER QUARTER FOR CODERS: 2015-2016

	First Quarter 2015	Second Quarter 2015	Third Quarter 2015	Fourth Quarter 2015	First Quarter 2016	Second Quarter 2016	Third Quarter 2016	Fourth Quarter 2016
Mary	1.2390	1.2214	1.1376	1.1689	1.2135	1.1739	1.2108	1.2594
Andrew	1.2249	1.2003	1.2121	1.1329	1.2260	1.2157	1.2241	1.1998
Joan	1.2423	1.3151	1.2971	1.2455	1.2646	1.2439	1.2876	1.2321
Frances	X	X	X					
Facility CMI Avg	1.2354	1.2456	1.2156	1.4354	1.4141	1.4032	1.4056	1.4040

EXERCISE 7-2

Reimbursement Statistics

Use the table below to answer the following questions.

MS-DRG	PATIENT DISCHARGES	RELATIVE WEIGHT	WEIGHT TOTAL
039 – Extracranial Procedures W/O CC/MCC	88	1.0452	
057 – Degenerative Nervous System Disorders W/O MCC	71	0.9841	
064 – Intracranial Hemorrhage or Cerebral Infarction W MCC	70	1.7417	
065 – Intracranial Hemorrhage or Cerebral Infarction W CC	69	1.0776	
066 – Intracranial Hemorrhage or Cerebral Infarction W/O CC/MCC	50	0.7566	
069 – Transient Ischemia	50	0.6948	
074 – Cranial & Peripheral Nerve Disorders W/O MCC	48	0.8786	
101 – Seizures W/O MCC	46	0.7569	
149 – Dysequilibrium	43	0.6184	
176 – Pulmonary Embolism W/O MCC	42	0.9891	
177 – Respiratory Infections & Inflammations W MCC	37	1.9934	
178 – Respiratory Infections & Inflammations W CC	29	1.3955	
189 – Pulmonary Edema & Respiratory Failure	18	1.2184	

1. What is the total weight for these MS-DRGs?

2. What is this hospital's CMI?

EXERCISE 7-2
Reimbursement Statistics—cont'd

3. Given the number of discharges and total weights below, calculate the case mix index for each month.

MONTH	DISCHARGES	TOTAL WEIGHT	CMI
January	2331	8355.49281	
February	2646	8819.9118	
March	2100	6757.3800	
April	2191	6483.1690	
May	2520	7270.2000	
June	1946	5424.2804	
July	1806	5618.6466	
August	2520	7572.6000	
September	2800	8396.3600	
October	2408	7192.9368	
November	2877	9104.2665	
December	2863	9417.5522	

COMPLIANCE STATISTICS

The Health Information Management Department may be asked for a variety of types of data and statistics for accreditation purposes. These can include incomplete or **delinquent record counts**—those past the allowed 30 day after discharge completion window—or other quality measures based on the contents of the medical record. Incomplete items may include nondictated or transcribed reports, or lack of signatures for those reports. The Joint Commission (TJC) allows a delinquent record count of 50%, or half the average number of hospital discharges, based on a **rolling quarterly average**, which is a way of calculating the average for the previous three months (one quarter of the year) with each passing month. For example, if the average discharges are 1500 per month for the first three months of January, February, and March, the next three months in the rolling quarter are February, March, and April. By looking at the rolling quarterly average, the HIM director is regularly updating the maximum allowed number of delinquent records. This is updated based on hospital discharge activity monthly. In this manner, the quarter rolls throughout the year and consists of the prior three months for which you have full discharge data.

Calculating delinquent record counts is relatively simple and involves averages of discharge data for a facility. Once the average is determined, it is then multiplied by 0.5 to determine the allowable number of incomplete records in a quarter, 50%. The table below shows the calculation of the allowed delinquent records for each month of one rolling quarter. In the hospital, the discharges and number of delinquent records would be provided based on hospital data.

Delinquent record count The number of records not completed within a specific time frame, such as within 30 days of discharge.

TJC The Joint Commission.

Rolling quarterly average The average of the previous three months.

Month	Number of Discharges	Rolling Quarterly Average (Add the Previous Three Months' Discharges, then Divide by 3)	Allowed Delinquent Records (50% of Rolling Quarterly Average)	Number of Delinquent Records
January	1761	$\dfrac{1761 + 1558 + 1802}{3} = 1707$	$1707 \times 0.5 = 853.5 = 854$	903
February	1558	$\dfrac{1761 + 1558 + 1802}{3} = 1707$	$1707 \times 0.5 = 853.5 = 854$	822
March	1802	$\dfrac{1761 + 1558 + 1802}{3} = 1707$	$1707 \times 0.5 = 853.5 = 854$	850

For January, this facility is over the allowed amount of delinquent records because 903 is greater than the allowed amount of 854. An HIM director might attribute this to the holidays or flu season, but nevertheless, it would need to be reported to The Joint Commission.

A more strict measure of performance might be History and Physical (H&P) completion within 24 hours of admission. The information contained in the H&P (Figure 7-3) is vital for patient care and utilization review, and case management so that the compliance rate is closely monitored. Let us look a little closer at the H&P requirement. This delinquency rate should be quite low but varies by facility. If we use the same discharge data as in the prior example but an allowable delinquency rate of only 2%, our calculations would be as follows:

H&P History and Physical.

Month	Number of Discharges	Rolling Quarterly Average (Add the Previous 3 Months' Discharges, then Divide by 3)	Allowed Delinquent H&Ps (2% of Rolling Quarterly Average)	Number of Delinquent H&Ps
January	1761	$\dfrac{1761 + 1558 + 1802}{3} = 1707$	$1707 \times 0.02 = 34.14 = 34$	28
February	1558	$\dfrac{1761 + 1558 + 1802}{3} = 1707$	$1707 \times 0.02 = 34.14 = 34$	29
March	1802	$\dfrac{1761 + 1558 + 1802}{3} = 1707$	$1707 \times 0.02 = 34.14 = 34$	36

As in the prior example, the number of discharges and number of delinquent H&Ps are provided based on hospital data, but the averages and allowable delinquent H&Ps are being calculated. In this hospital for January and February, the physicians provided H&Ps within 24 hours more than 98% of the time. In March, however, the physicians were not in compliance with this requirement because more than 34 H&Ps were not completed within the 24-hour required time frame. When H&Ps are not available shortly after admission, case management nurses cannot quickly plan for services needed on discharge of certain patients.

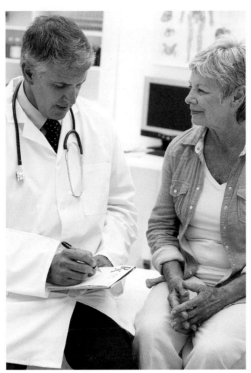

Figure 7-3 The information contained in the History and Physical (H&P) is vital for care both while the patient is in the hospital and following discharge.

EXERCISE 7-3
Accreditation Statistics

1. You just received the discharge data for last month, July. What three months should be included in the rolling quarterly average?

   Use the following discharge data from a rural hospital to perform your calculations.

Month	Discharges
January	333
February	378
March	300
April	313
May	360
June	278
July	258
August	360
September	400
October	344
November	411
December	409

2. Calculate the average patient discharges for February, March, and April.

3. How many delinquent records are allowed if the most recent month for which you have discharge data is November?

4. How many missing H&P reports can you have for each month of a rolling quarter ending in September? How many H&P reports can be missing the next month, with a rolling quarter ending in October?

REVIEW QUESTIONS

1. You expect your scanners to produce 1800 images per hour. Assuming the scanners work full time for a year with no time off, how many images would they be expected to produce in a year? If 3 weeks are taken for vacation and holidays, how many images should they produce? If a push rate is given of 2000 images per hour, how does this latter calculation differ?

2. Transcriptionist B produced 222,000 lines last year. He/she works 32 hours per week, or a maximum of 1664 hours per year. He/she took 3 days off for vacation, 5 days off for holidays, and 8 days off for sick time. What would his/her total number of productive days be (keep in mind that he/she works 4 days a week)? What is his/her daily production of transcription lines?

3. If it takes 15 minutes to code one inpatient record and your facility had 1558 discharges in February, how many hours would it take to code the records? How many FTEs does this equate to?

4. Coders at your facility are expected to code three inpatient charts per hour. In March, your facility discharged 1802 patients. How many full-time inpatient coders would be needed to complete the coding of these records? (Remember, with FTEs, you cannot round up or down much, so it may be necessary to hire a part-time employee!)

5. It takes 20 minutes to prepare one inpatient record for ROI. The department staffs Jenna full-time, and Clare works 4 hours a day in the afternoons, 5 days a week. How many requests can they fulfill in a day?

6. The Medicare case mix index for March at Happy Valley Community Hospital was reported as 2.1326. You are asked to verify this given the total weight of all DRGs of 2915.2882 and the number of Medicare discharges as 1567. Can you verify the Medicare case mix index report? At St. Barnabus, the case mix index is 1.5719. What is the difference between the case mix index at the two hospitals?

7. Your facility has reported discharges for the past quarter as follows: March 1802; April 1959; May 1972. You are working on your Joint Commission statistics and need to calculate the average monthly discharges for this quarter. Once you have completed that, you must then calculate your allowable delinquent chart amount and your allowable delinquent H&P amount. What are these three numbers?

FINANCIAL DATA

CHAPTER OUTLINE

BUDGETING OVERVIEW
CAPITAL BUDGET
   Payback Period

Return on Investment
Renting or Leasing Equipment

OPERATIONAL BUDGET
   Variance
REVIEW QUESTIONS

KEY TERMS

accrual accounting
amortization
capital budget
cash flow

depreciation
fixed cost
operational budget
payback period

return on investment (ROI)
variable cost
variance

LEARNING OBJECTIVES

At the end of the chapter, you should be able to do the following:

1. Distinguish between a capital and an operational budget.
2. Calculate return on investment (ROI) and the payback period for a capital expenditure.

3. Demonstrate understanding of monthly budgets and budget variances.

Each one of us must make sure the money we earn covers our monthly bills and expenses; we should also think to the future and save extra money for large items, like a house or a car. If you are well organized, you might even have a budget that you use to proportion out your money each month and gauge your success in meeting these financial goals. Similarly, each department in a hospital is expected to operate within the financial constraints provided by a budget.

BUDGETING OVERVIEW

Budgets are based on a fiscal year, which may or may not be the same as a calendar year. For example, fiscal years may start on July 1 and end on June 30 or may start on October 1 and end on September 30. Budgets are a tool for facilities to plan for **cash flow**, the balance of money in and money out of the department. Therefore, each department within a hospital or clinic is required to follow a budget and must plan for purchases on a timeline provided (in a specific month). This will ensure that the facility has the funds to pay for an item when a purchase is made.

○ **Cash flow** The balance of money in and money out of the department.

TAKE AWAY ●·········

A budget ensures the facility or department has enough money to pay for its expenses.

BRIEF CASE

WORKING WITH THE BUDGET

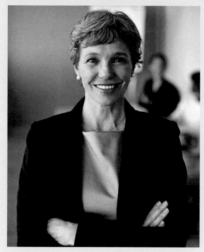

Kate, an HIM director, is required to participate in hospital-wide budget plans every fall for the upcoming fiscal year beginning July 1st. She must also plan for future technology enhancements to satisfy the facility's meaningful use goals, a set of measures set by Centers for Medicare and Medicaid (CMS) that rewards providers for adopting new technologies. Successfully implementing Electronic Health Record (EHR) technologies will result in nearly $40,000 in additional incentive payments from Medicaid and Medicaid over the next three years, as well reducing the time and money lost from rejected claims.

○ **CMS** Centers for Medicare and Medicaid.

○ **EHR** Electronic Health Record.

Remember, there are many different departments in a hospital, each having unique financial demands. Many of these departments are competing for funds at the same time. To help the facility with future financial plans, including fair and proper allocation of funds, each department must submit annual proposals for two kinds of budgets: the *capital budget*, for large, one-time purchases, and the *operational budget*, for daily operations.

How does the facility determine the amount of money available to spend? In Chapter 7, we discussed case mix index (CMI, an average of the type of patients a facility treats). Although this can change over time, the CMI does give the Chief Financial Officer (CFO) an idea of anticipated revenue. This provides a starting point for budgetary plans as an indicator of the revenues the facility will make based on the patients treated in the past.

Health Information Management (HIM) is not directly involved in billing and collections, and it is typically not considered to be a revenue-producing department. The exception to this is if release of information (ROI) is done in-house, and a revenue stream is generated from that source. The budget concerns of the HIM director revolve around expenses and, therefore, use **accrual accounting**. This simply means that the budget records expenses for

○ **CMI** Case mix index.

○ **CFO** Chief financial officer.

○ **HIM** Health Information Management.

○ **ROI** Release of information.

items anticipated in specific months, regardless of when the expense was actually paid. Say, for example, the AHIMA conference takes place in October. Even though the department would purchase plane tickets and hotel accommodations a month or more ahead of time, those expenses are recorded for the month of October. The payment of various expenses will likely occur both before and after the actual date of the meeting, but using accrual accounting, we budget for the entire amount in one month, October.

CAPITAL BUDGET

Capital budget expenditures are large purchases, such as equipment. Each facility defines what constitutes a capital expense by the dollar amount value. For example, some facilities may consider anything over $1000 as a capital expenditure, while others may define this as $5000 or more. HIM department directors must think carefully about what they will need in the future in terms of new equipment and/or technology.

The cost for such items is not only the price of the new equipment. Considerations for these major expenditures must also take into account the training needed to use the equipment and/or technology. This expense may be included in the purchase price, but additional training time should be considered. Paid training can become costly, but adequate training of personnel prior to a "go live"—the day the new equipment is put into service—is essential to a successful outcome. In addition, service contracts to update and maintain the equipment and/or technology must also be considered. These may not be optional and can be rather costly.

Often, projections for capital purchases are required three to five years (or even longer) prior to the purchase. This can be challenging, and it is helpful to attend annual meetings such as the AHIMA conference, to see what vendors are offering now or planning to offer. Also, networking among HIM professionals is useful to see what they are doing now or planning to do in the future.

Payback Period

When a capital equipment request is submitted, justification for the expense is required (Fig. 8-1). *Why do we need to make this purchase, and how will it help the department do its job?* Financial justifications can be required in the form of a **payback period**, which determines how long it will take to recover the expense of the equipment. To calculate the payback period, the numerator is the total cost of the equipment, and the denominator is the estimated cash inflow resulting from use of the new equipment.

 Calculating the Payback Period

$$\text{Payback period} = \frac{\text{Cost of equipment}}{\text{Estimated cash inflow}}$$

For example, a department might consider buying a new scanner to digitize health records. The model that best meets its needs has a sticker price of $6300, and a four-year maintenance agreement costs an additional $1200. The initial cost of the scanner is $7500. But with this new technology, the department gets higher quality scans and fewer rescans, amounting to monthly savings of $250, or annual savings estimated at $3000. The payback period would therefore be calculated as follows:

$$\text{Payback period} = \frac{\$7500}{\$3000} = \frac{5}{2} = 2.5 \text{ years or 2 years and six months}$$

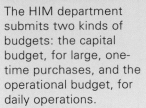

Accrual accounting an accounting method in which income and expenses are recorded when they are incurred, regardless of when the money is actually exchanged.

TAKE AWAY

The HIM department submits two kinds of budgets: the capital budget, for large, one-time purchases, and the operational budget, for daily operations.

Capital budget money set aside for larger purchases, usually over a certain dollar amount whose use will span multiple fiscal years.

TAKE AWAY

When considering purchases, all fees, down payments, and add-on charges must be considered so that you are choosing the best option for your facility.

Payback period the amount of time it will take for the savings or revenues generated by a purchase to pay for the purchase.

Description _____   Budget Year _____
                                        Budget Cost $ _____
Manufacturer _____   Unity Cost _____
                                        Quantity _____
Model # _____   Total _____
                                        Freight _____
Vendor _____   Installation _____
                                        Quorum Discount _____
Materials Manager Signature _____   TOTAL COST $ _____

1. Type of expenditure: Replacement _____   New _____

2. Briefly define function of capital expenditure _____
_____
_____

3. Estimate # of procedures to be done _____   **4.** Average charge per procedure _____

5. Will the number of FTE's increase or decrease _____   **6.** By how many _____

7. Briefly describe why item is needed _____
_____
_____
_____
_____

8. Financial analysis   Annual   **REQUESTED BY:**

    a. Gross revenue $ _____   _____
    b. Less: Salaries   _____   Department Director   Date
    c.   Supplies   _____
    d.   Depreciation   _____
    e.   Professional fees   _____
    f.   Other (itemize) _____   _____   **APPROVED BY:**
    g.   _____   _____
    h.   _____   _____
    i.   (Total sum b-h)   _____   Dept. Asst. Administrator   Date
    j. Gross profit (a-i)   _____
    k. Less: Contractual adjustments   _____
    l.   Bad debts   _____   Maintenance Director   Date
    m. Policy discounts   _____
    n.   Total (sum k-m)   _____
    o. Gross margin (j-n) $ _____   Asst. Admin.—Finance   Date
    p. Asset cost   _____
    q. Return in investment   _____ %
    r. Payback period   _____   Administrator   Date

Figure 8-1 Capital expenditure approval form. (From: Huron Regional Medical Center, Huron, SD, USA.)

Depending on the circumstances, that payback period may be too long. If the expected life of the equipment is five years, then a shorter payback period, such as one to two years, is likely preferred. If the facility requires a one-year payback period, then the HIM manager may need to look to other ways to meet this goal, such as a less expensive piece of equipment or a lease plan, rather than purchase.

Return on investment The percentage of the capital expenditure recovered each year.

Return on Investment

Another way to look at the value of capital equipment purchases is **return on investment (ROI)**, which represents how much of the equipment cost is recovered per year.

Stat Tip ·····································

Watch out for context! The abbreviation ROI is most often used in the field of health information management to mean *release of information*, which is the HIM department function of disclosing patient health information. However, in business, ROI is also a commonly used abbreviation for *return on investment*. Since health care is a business, HIM professionals will encounter both usages of the abbreviation ROI on the job.

Return on investment is calculated with the average annual savings as the numerator over the purchase price, multiplied by 100 to get a percentage.

 Calculating Return on Investment

$$\text{Return on investment} = \frac{\text{Average annual savings}}{\text{Purchase price}} \times 100$$

Let us plug the numbers for the new scanner into the formula to find out how quickly the equipment pays itself off. We estimated that the scanner would save $250 per month, or $3000 annually:

$$\frac{\$3000}{\$7500} \times 100 = 40\% \text{ return on investment}$$

In other words, 40% of the scanner is paid off after one year and 80% after two years. If the facility has a required minimum return on investment, such as 35%, then the new scanner would be considered a good investment. We might think about this return on investment as how quickly we are getting the money back that we put into it. After we reach 100% ROI, we are making a profit on our investment; we continue to save money each month but have already paid for the piece of equipment.

Renting or Leasing Equipment

A facility may choose to pay for a large purchase monthly rather than as an initial lump sum. Renting or leasing shifts the cost of the purchase from the capital budget to the operational budget. Rather than purchasing the scanner outright, renting for a year and then purchasing the scanner may be considered. If rental cost (plus maintenance) is $350 per month, then the cost to the department annually is $4200 ($350 × 12). Although the monthly cost is higher than an outright purchase, renting allows for more frequently updated technology and the advantage of not being stuck with outdated technology after the equipment is paid off. Additionally, if the option exists to apply part of the rental expense to a future purchase (for example, 50% of this or $2100), renting can become a much more attractive option.

A third option might be a lease, such as you might choose for a car. Consider a required four-year contract at a cost of $300 per month. Although less than renting per month, this will add up to $3600 annually. At the end of four years, the department will have paid a total of $14,400. This is almost double the purchase price of the scanner and well past the original payback period for the equipment. So, what makes renting or leasing compelling? Why would anyone do this if the monthly savings from the new equipment purchase is $250, while the monthly lease cost is $300? Renting or leasing offers the chance to update the technology, and equipment companies often offer those sweeteners to buy. In addition, some departments just do not have the initial outlay of money needed to buy the equipment outright.

The table below compares the cost of purchasing, renting, and leasing. These three options can be combined, such as a lease- or rent-to-purchase arrangement, and an

HIM department manager must consider each carefully, with his or her overall budget and goals in mind.

	Purchase *(48-Month Amortization)*	Rent *(Short-Term, 12 Months)*	Lease *(Long-Term, 48 Months)*
Monthly expense including maintenance	$156.25	$350	$300
Total	**$7500**	**$4200 per year**	**$14,400**

> ## Stat Tip ···
>
> Initial quotes might seem advantageous, but careful calculations on a per-month or even per-copy (or scan) basis may show that the least expensive option requires a higher volume than your facility produces.

As you can see, obtaining equipment takes planning, and options for payment should be considered with the facility CFO. If new technology is consistently being introduced, then purchasing an expensive piece of equipment may not be the best answer. The department may want to rent for a year and then purchase the newer technology. These various options also impact budget reports, of course, since monthly allocations from the operational budget are required for renting or leasing. In addition, even if the department purchases the scanner outright, it may choose to *amortize* the cost of the capital equipment over several years to represent the actual projected life of the equipment. **Amortization** finances the purchase with a fixed payment schedule of principal and interest over the life of a loan. This would also show as a monthly fixed cost, rather than a one-time capital expense on your budget report.

This monthly cost is also known as depreciation expense, which is a common practice in accrual-based accounting. Very few material items *appreciate* (gain value), but most do, indeed, **depreciate** (lose value) as they age. You may have heard the example of how a new car depreciates several thousand dollars the moment it is driven off of the dealer's lot. Straight-line depreciation is calculated by devaluing the initial cost by the number of years that the item is projected to be used. For example, a high-capacity printer that costs $2500 and has an expected use of 5 years will depreciate $500 each year ($2500 ÷ 5 years = $500). The first year, it is worth $2500; the second year, $2000; by the third year it is valued at $1500, the fourth $1000, and the fifth $500. After the fifth year, the printer's expected useful life has expired.

Amortization A fixed payment schedule of principal and interest over the life of a loan.

Depreciation The loss of value over time due to wear from use and obsolescence.

EXERCISE 8-1

Capital Budget

1. If an HIM department considers purchasing a high-volume/high-speed scanner for $18,000 that would save the department $500 a month, what is the ROI after one year?

2. What is the payback period for a piece of equipment that cost $6000 and saves $250 per month?

3. Using straight-line depreciation, how much would an $8800 piece of equipment depreciate each year on a 4-year depreciation schedule?

Health Information Management Department FY 2016 Budget

Salaries (8 FTEs)	325,498
Supplies	102,822
Equipment Leases	34,781
Equipment Rental	3,476
Equipment Depreciation	16,902
Outsourcing	12,441
Travel	1,542
Education	2,305
Dues/credentials	1,790
Total	501,557

Figure 8-2 A sample budget.

OPERATIONAL BUDGET

Operational budgets include routine expenditures, such as the equipment leases and maintenance contracts discussed above (Fig. 8-2). They also plan for payroll, office supplies, and even travel to conferences. Some of these expenditures would be **fixed costs**, such as the price of a lease for equipment (assuming this is a flat rate and not based on amount of usage). In the preparation of a budget, the fixed costs are the easiest to fill in since they are based on a contracted amount between the vendor and the facility. **Variable costs** can change depending on level of activity or volume. If the facility performs all release of information functions in-house, for example, then the postage and supply expense varies depending on the number of requests processed. Variable costs are estimated based on the prior year activity levels, along with any expected changes for the coming year. For example, if the capital budget includes the installation of new speech recognition software, then the payroll budget will not be identical to the previous year. The HIM manager would consider the added payroll for training and perhaps add in usage of a transcription vendor for two months while the staff adjusts to the new system.

Operational budget Costs related to the operation of the department, such as payroll, utilities, and supplies.

Fixed costs Expenses in the operational budget that do not change on a monthly basis.

Variable costs Expenses in the operational budget that change month to month based on the volume of activity.

Variance

After the operational budget is created and in place (usually a year ahead of time), the department director reports on *variances* from the budget, usually on a monthly basis. A **variance** is a deviation from the original prediction of what would be spent and when. These can be positive, meaning you spent less than predicted, or negative, meaning you spent more than predicted. Therefore, once the fiscal year begins, monthly budget results are examined. Even though some actual monthly expenditures may be above budgeted amounts (negative variance), hopefully some months will be below the budgeted amounts (positive variance), so the annual budget will be close to the initial target prediction.

For example, in a small facility, if an employee has an extended illness or injury, the unexpected cost of a temporary employee or outsourcing service may cause the payroll portion of the budget to show negative variance.

TAKE AWAY

Variable costs in the operational budget are estimated from the previous year's budget.

Variance A deviation from the projected spending in the budget.

	January	February	March	April	May	Total Budget	Variance
Danielle (out sick)	$2000 (sick time)	$2000 (vacation time)	$0	$0	$0	$10,000	$6000
Carol	$4000 ($1000 overtime to cover Danielle)	$3000	$3000	$3000	$3000	$15,000	($1000)
Outsourcing	$0	$3000	$3000	$2500	$2250		($10,750)
Variance	Over $1000	Over $3000	Over $1000	Over $500	Over $250		Over $5750

The above table shows that with Danielle out sick, the department needed assistance from an outsourcing company although they initially relied on overtime to cover the extra work. Eventually more of Danielle's responsibilities were able to be absorbed into other employees' routines, so the monthly amount for outsourcing diminished. However, after five months, the budget showed a negative variance of $5750 for these expenses.

The payroll portion of an operating budget is usually the highest percentage of the costs. The budget will likely require inclusion of fringe benefits at a rate of around 30%, which includes payroll taxes and vacation, holiday, and sick pay. If the facility provides annual reviews at the same time for all employees, then payroll projections for all raises can be made in the operating budget beginning in the same month.

For example, if all employee evaluations are done by September 1st and raises are based on performance (such as 3% for an above-average evaluation), then the adjustment in salary might begin on October 1st for all affected employees. When preparing the budget, assuming the fiscal year begins on July 1st, the HIM director would annualize the salaries for each month, then adjust once raises go into effect on October 1st. Each month, other expenditures to date can be annualized in a similar fashion by adding up the preceding months and dividing the total expenditures for each category by the total months to date. Then that average monthly figure can be used for each of the remaining months to see how far off the original projections were. The actual budget figures do not change, but as a manager, you have a more up-to-date picture of your expenditures for comparison.

For example, if an employee earns $24,000, then the annualized amount prior to a raise in pay would be $2000 per month. If a 3% increase occurs, then an additional $720 $(24,000 \times 0.03)$ would be added to the annual salary and divided by 12. The new monthly pay amount would then be $2060 for that employee beginning with the October 1st payroll. The HIM director would adjust the budget for these payroll increases as follows:

	August	September	October	November
Danielle	$2000	$2000	$2060	$2060
Carol	$3000	$3000	$3090	$3090
Jade	$3500	$3500	$3605	$3605
Karyn	$2800	$2800	$2884	$2884
Monthly payroll total	**$11,300**	**$11,300**	**$11,639**	**$11,639**

If a facility begins providing a new service, such as heart catheterizations, the HIM department should consider additional transcription and coding services at a minimum. It will need additional staff until its current staff is able to keep up with the volume of new cases and acquire the new skills needed to properly complete reports and provide codes for these services. Rather than hiring additional staff in this situation, many HIM directors would pay the existing staff overtime or hire an outsourcing company to assist temporarily with the extra work. Using current employees may be optimal since they will be more familiar with the physicians and work types. However, too much overtime can lead to errors and exhaustion, so these factors must be weighed in this decision. An outsourcing company should be able to quickly get up to speed with the demands and provide the extra resources needed. However, these resources can be more expensive than overtime expenses.

Conversely, sometimes there are declines in patient volume, and health care facilities are required to cut staff or hours. Ideally, this is done by *attrition*, which means that positions are not filled when they are vacated. However, sometimes hours must be cut to avoid letting staff go. In this case, an HIM department director may be asked to cut hourly employees to a 32-hour work week from a 40-hour work week. Some jobs may be eliminated altogether. These are difficult decisions that must be undertaken with a great deal of research and forethought. It is important to remember the time and effort the facility has invested in the training of these highly skilled workers.

EXERCISE 8-2
Operational Budget

1. The HIM department pays $22 each month for a firm to remove, shred, and recycle its paper waste securely. In May, the cost per month will raise to $25 per month. Is this a fixed cost or a variable cost?

2. Including benefits, you pay Mindy $2600 a month. Are Mindy's wages fixed or variable?

3. Mindy's salary (including benefits) is $31,200, and she received a 3 on her performance review, meaning her work "Meets Expectations." She will receive a 1% raise in May. Maddox makes the same amount per year, but her score of 1, "Meets and Frequently Exceeds Expectations," will earn her a 5% raise. What is the payroll budget for these two employees for May?

BRIEF CASE

PREPARING A REQUEST FOR PROPOSAL (RFP)

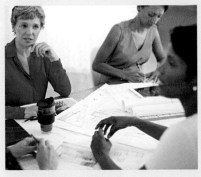

Kate's facility has recently acquired a large physician practice, and after careful review, her coding manager recommends that an EHR be used to improve efficiency and accuracy of submitted claims for these physicians. Due to turnover and training issues, the returned claims were about 5% of total submissions last year (300,000 claims). The accuracy standards require 98.5% accuracy, and she hopes to see this standard applied enterprise-wide for all coding.

The EHR salesman states that the new system will improve completeness of submitted claims, thereby reducing the returned claims by 80%. If the salesman is correct, Kate could potentially decrease the staff who follow up on these claims by 1.5 FTE, which is an annual savings of about $39,000 (including benefits). In reality, this may be a low estimate of annual savings because of improved efficiency and better turnaround of claims processing. The cost of the EHR under consideration for the group practice will be $106,000. Help Kate justify the capital purchase by answering the following questions:

1. How many claims were returned last year?

2. What does the standard (98.5%) allow for returned claims?

3. According to the salesman, will the encoder meet the accuracy standard?

4. What is the payback period?

5. What is the return on investment (ROI)?

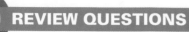

REVIEW QUESTIONS

1. Explain the difference between the operational budget and the capital budget, giving examples of the types of expenses in each.

2. You sent out five RFPs (requests for proposals) to compare costs and benefits of a new copy machine. You only received two of the RFPs back. The first, Reliable Copier Company, gives you a cost of $3800, which includes a 5-year maintenance contract of $1500. The cost savings per month for this first proposal is projected at $150. The second proposal from Kwick Kopy Services is at a cost of $4100 with a 5-year maintenance contract of $800 included and a cost savings per month of $100. Which payback period is quicker?

3. You realize the department will need a new scanner in three years, so you anticipate the purchase price of a scanner in three years based on quotes from three of your sales representatives. As time passes, you realize this may need to be adjusted based on budgetary restrictions or new technology, but you are comfortable budgeting $8400, and you prepare a justification report to go along with the capital budget request. The hospital is asking for a 35% ROI in the first year for a purchase, otherwise you will need to consider renting or leasing. Given the following information, which option should you choose?

	ScanTron	ScanTek	Scans 'R' Us
Price	$7900	$8400	$6500
Savings per month	$225	$275	$180
ROI			

4. Examine the following annual budget variance report and double-check the calculations. If available, use an Excel spreadsheet and embedded formulas for calculations. The "Budget" and "Actual" columns are correct, but are there any errors in the $Var or %Var columns? Based on this report, how would you change the budget for next year?

Item	Budget	Actual	$Var	%Var
Payroll	$1,560,000	$1,555,555	$4555	0.28%
Outsourcing	$5000	$10,750	($5750)	115%
Supplies	$3500	$3000	$500	12.4%
AHIMA dues and credentials	$2220	$2405	($85)	(8.3%)
Equipment depreciation	$3750	$3750	0	100%
Equipment lease	$7200	$6000	$1200	0.16%
Equipment rental	$700	$1400	$700	(100%)

ADVANCED DATA ANALYSIS TECHNIQUES

SCRUBBING AND MAPPING DATA

CHAPTER OUTLINE

KEY TERMS

data accuracy
data cleansing
data comprehensiveness
data consistency
data constraints

data dictionary
data enhancement
data harmonization
data mapping
data scrubbing

heuristics
master patient index (MPI)
source
target

LEARNING OBJECTIVES

At the conclusion of this chapter, you should be able to do the following:

1. Explain the importance of data quality and define the characteristics of quality data.
2. Define data scrubbing terminology.
3. Analyze a data set for data cleansing issues.
4. Define data mapping terminology.
5. Evaluate a mapped data set for errors.

INTRODUCTION

So far in your study, you have learned how to analyze and present data that has been collected for a hospital system or physician practice. Although it might sound like common sense, the data collected is not useful if it is wrong. Our bassinet count, for example, is meaningless if it includes a 75-year-old patient. The autopsy rate will not be useful if there are negative numbers in our counts. The Cesarean section rate will not tell us anything if there are men in the denominator. In particular, we want to make sure our data is complete, consistent, and accurate. We want to make sure we are using quality data.

BRIEF CASE

WORKING WITH QUALITY DATA

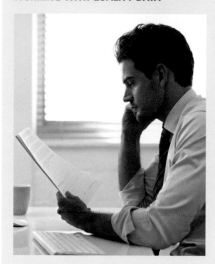

Hector a new data analyst for a large physician practice, is in the process of reviewing survey results from a recent study. "Hindsight is 20/20," he says to himself looking at the printout. One of the questions at the end of the survey was an add-on, asking for the responder's zip code. He could see that there were 5-digit and 9-digit zip codes, blanks, and illegible entries. And then there were what appeared to be multiple surveys from patients with the same name. He is going to have to fix this if she wants to be able to use the data!

DATA QUALITY

DQM Data quality model.

AHIMA American health information management association.

Data accuracy A data quality characteristic ensuring data are correct, valid, and free from errors.

Data comprehensiveness A data quality characteristic ensuring all required data are collected.

In the Data Quality Model (DQM), the American Health Information Management Association (AHIMA) identifies specific dimensions of what constitutes quality data, listed in Table 9-1.[1] Our discussion will focus on three of these characteristics: *accuracy*, *comprehensiveness*, and *consistency*.

- **Data accuracy** is a measure of the true values that exist. You will need to check that the data is actually correct. Your data needs to be validated by checking for the absence of impossible entries. For example, are the patients who carry delivery codes always women? Are men the only patients who undergo prostatectomies? Are you treating patients who have birth dates after 1900? Do you have valid addresses and zip codes? Do you have code numbers that exist?
- **Data comprehensiveness** ensures you have all of the data included that are needed for the task at hand. Do your data require an address that is a street, city, and zip code? Are all of those elements present? If not, is it because the data is missing? For example, a patient may not have responded to the question regarding their religious affiliation. The column could then be completed with a "missing data" field, and in the future, an option for no response given can be added.

---

[1] AHIMA. "Data Quality Management Model (Updated)." Journal of AHIMA 83, no.7 (July 2012): 62–67.

TABLE 9-1

DATA QUALITY CHARACTERISTICS

CHARACTERISTIC	DEFINITION	EXAMPLES
Accuracy	Data are correct, valid, and free from errors.	ICD codes are actual codes that are correct for the documentation. The patient's names and DOB are correctly recorded.
Accessibility	Data items are easily and legally obtainable.	Name, DOB, admission and discharge dates are all easy to collect, *and* only those who are legally allowed to view the data are able to.
Comprehensiveness	All required data items are collected.	The entire data of birth is collected, not just the year and month.
Consistency	Data are reliable and the same.	Temperatures are recorded as either Fahrenheit or Celsius, but not both. The month of discharge is recorded as two digits.
Currency	Data are up to date.	Diagnoses and procedures are coded with the then current coding system.
Data definition	The meaning of a healthcare-related data element.	Blood pressure is the recording of systolic over diastolic pressure.
Granularity	Data are at the correct level of detail.	Lab values for an A1c are recorded with one decimal place (not as whole numbers).
Precision	Data values are just large enough to support the application or process with acceptable limits defined.	Pulse and respirations are recorded as whole numbers.
Relevancy	Data are meaningful to the performance of the process for which they are collected.	Blood pressure data before and after medication change is a relevant use of data. Use of temperature would not be useful.
Timeliness	Timeliness is determined by how the data are being used and their context.	Timely data collection of average blood sugar levels through the use of an A1c would be every three months; whereas daily monitoring gives a singular reading.

- **Data consistency** means the data is reliable and in the same format. Are the data the same across different databases, and if not, which is the correct data? For example, patients may use different names, telephone numbers, contacts, or insurance information at different physician practices. If the databases are to be merged in order to be statistically analyzed, the most recent, "true" values need to be found. An old telephone number will not be useful when trying to contact a patient, when a newer number is the one that should be used.

A perfect example of the need for data quality can be illustrated by the need for consistency in a **master patient index (MPI)**. An MPI is a database of all the patients who have received care at a facility, along with their encounter information, and is often used to correlate the patient with the file identification. Essentially, patients have an all-too-human tendency to use slightly different information (names, addresses, phone numbers, etc.) when seeking health care. Imagine, for example, a patient named

Data consistency A data quality characteristic ensuring data are reliable and the same.

Master patient index (MPI) A system containing a list of patients who have received care at the health care facility and their encounter information, often used to correlate the patient with the file identification.

Jonathon Thomas Langley, Jr. When seeking care on one occasion, he may give his full name; on another, he may sign in as Jon rather than Jonathon, omit the suffix Jr., use only his middle initial T rather than spelling out Thomas, or any combination of the above. A complete and accurate MPI maintained with data quality ensures those differences in Mr. Langley's name are resolved to properly identify the patient for future visits or admissions.

Stat Tip

While most of the fields are either alpha or numeric, some hospitals are even using palm scans to verify identity because patients give different information every time they come to the emergency room.

BRIEF CASE

USING QUALITY DATA

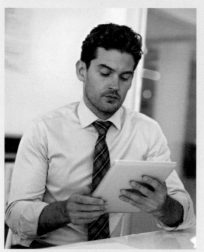

For part of the survey, Hector must compare data for two different physicians regarding patient length of stay for a variety of diagnoses. Other variables include sex, age, religious preference, and patient zip code. As he scans the data, he notices some problems. What type of issue is each of the following?

1. The list of diagnoses for one of the physicians appears to have patients who were also treated by the opposite physician. While this may be true, he notices that 10 of the patients appear to be the same but have different addresses. This is an issue of data _____.

2. One of the patients, Michael McCarthy, lives on 701 March Rd., Norcross, Georgia. His zip code is listed as 30003. Hector notices another patient whose address is 1155 March Rd., with the same city and state, but whose zip code is listed as 30030-0003. What data quality problems does he see?

○ **Data dictionary** A list of details that describe each field in a database.

TAKE AWAY ○·········

A data dictionary helps maintain data quality by defining exactly what should be entered into a database and how it should be entered.

We can ensure the quality of our data using what is called a data dictionary. A **data dictionary** is a list of details that describe each field in a database and dictates how the information needs to be recorded (Fig. 9-1). These include descriptors of each data element giving the limitations of characters, numbers, length of the field, and any limitations as to their use. For example, the field in the database for the patient's last name might be limited to 12 characters. The admission date field may be eight numbers separated by forward slashes. Any use of numbers in the first example, or characters in the second, would be considered errors according to the confines of the data dictionary. Looking again at the list of data quality characteristics in Table 9-1, which characteristics do you think are encouraged by a proper data dictionary? By defining exactly what data must be collected and how, the data dictionary ensures the data is consistent, comprehensive, relevant, and recorded with the proper level of granularity.

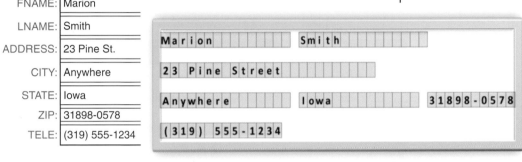

Name	Definition	Size	Type	Example
FNAME	Patient's first name	15 Characters	Alphabetic	Marion
LNAME	Patient's last name	15 Characters	Alphabetic	Smith
ADDRESS	Patient's home street address	25 Characters	Alphanumeric	23 Pine St
CITY	City associated with ADDRESS	15 Characters	Alphabetic	Anywhere
STATE	State associated with ADDRESS	14 Characters	Alphabetic	IOWA
ZIP	Postal zip code associated with ADDRESS	10 Characters	Alphanumeric	31898-0578
TELE	Patient's primary contact number	14 Characters	Alphanumeric	(319) 555-1234

FNAME: Marion
LNAME: Smith
ADDRESS: 23 Pine St.
CITY: Anywhere
STATE: Iowa
ZIP: 31898-0578
TELE: (319) 555-1234

Marion   Smith
23 Pine Street
Anywhere   Iowa   31898-0578
(319) 555-1234

Each field in the record above is blocked to illustrate the number of characters allowed, compared to the number this record required.

Figure 9-1 The data dictionary defines exactly how data should be collected to maintain quality and use quality data.

EXERCISE 9-1

Data Quality

1. Which element of data quality is violated when temperatures are recorded as whole numbers instead of with one decimal place?

2. Which element of data quality ensures diagnoses and procedures in an inpatient setting are not coded with ICD-9-CM?

3. Which element of data quality is violated when only the diastolic pressure reading is recorded?

4. How does a data dictionary help ensure quality data?

DATA SCRUBBING

If data is not collected with the elements of data quality in mind, it needs to be cleaned before it can be useful. The process of cleaning up data for analysis is called **data cleansing** or **data scrubbing**. Let us begin with an example of data scrubbing. On closer inspection of the data, a patient record may be incomplete with missing data (gender, city, etc.), or the data might have been inconsistently recorded (5-digit vs. 9-digit zip codes), or there were duplicate records (two or more for the same patient), or perhaps even incorrect information (insurance information out of date or just plain wrong). As the saying states, "garbage in, garbage out," so cleaning up the data for analysis is necessary to get reliable (and useful!) results.

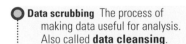

Data scrubbing The process of making data useful for analysis. Also called **data cleansing**.

The first step in cleaning data is to assign an individual who is responsible for overseeing the task. That person may be the database administrator or a health information or health services manager. The task is one that needs to be a maintenance function, routinely performed on a weekly or monthly basis on a patient database. If the data in question are from a study, such as survey results, then of course the cleaning is done before any analysis is performed; the responsibility for the cleaning is most likely the providence of the researcher.

After the data is collected and before it is cleaned, *the most important step is to back up the database.* This original copy needs to be labeled as such, dated, and kept separately. If, in the process of tidying up the errors and omissions, more errors and omissions are inadvertently created, the original is always available to rescue the effort.

Stat Tip ···

Always back up your original data and keep it separate from the file you are cleaning. This is your safety file if anything goes wrong. You will be grateful when things go wrong (and they will).

BRIEF CASE

SCRUBBING THE DATA

The inconsistent zip codes in Hector's survey could have been avoided with a proper data dictionary. Take a look at the zip codes collected below. Mark each entry that does not meet the standards of data accuracy, granularity, or consistency. Then, create a data dictionary for the zip code field to prevent this from happening in the future.

Last name	First name	Zip code
Anton	Mark	5899
Bahar	Allen	58991
Crawford	Sarah	58991-2344
Darden	Tawanna	589999
Endee	Robert	5899!
Frick	David	58923
George	Ivory	58832
Hu	Dallas	58992-33
Iwasaki	Thomas	058999
Jurawski	Geoffrey	58999-

DATA DICTIONARY
Patient Demographics

NAME	DEFINITION	SIZE	TYPE	EXAMPLE
FNAME	Patient's first name	15 Characters	Alphabetic	Geoffrey
LNAME	Patient's last name	15 Characters	Alphabetic	Jurawski
ZIP				58831

Data Constraints and Harmonization

The data dictionary works through the use of *data constraints*. **Data constraints** are rules that limit the type of data that can be entered into a field. For example, a *data-type constraint* would be whether the data is alpha or numeric. A patient's sex may be recorded as F for female or M for male. Then again, there may be a system of using O for female and 1 for male. The person responsible for reviewing data quality will have to be aware of the constraint on the particular data item. *Unique constraints* are those that occur only once per patient—like his/her medical record or social security number. A *mandatory constraint* is one that requires that a field must be filled in. An example would be a patient's name, date of birth, and/or medical record number. *Set-membership constraints* are those that restrict a data field to a given number of options: M (married), S (single), W (widowed), D (divorced), or P (partnered). No other options are allowed in the field. A *range constraint* is one that has limits as to a possible range. Patients could not have a date of birth, for example, before 1900 or beyond today's date. A *foreign-key constraint* is one that has a data field (column) of unique values that is shared with other databases. It could be a patient's zip code, date of discharge, or physician ID number. Each of these is unique but appears in several patient records. Because of that, a foreign-key constraint means that whatever the data is that is recorded, it must have a standardized format.

Other aspects of data scrubbing are **data harmonization**, which is the change of all short forms of words like Jr. or Sr., or St. or Rd., to their full length: Junior or Senior, Street or Road. Otherwise, an attempt at merging databases could result in duplication of records. **Data enhancement** is the activity of adding information by checking against a validated database. For example, by using the Social Security Death Match Master File, a database from the Social Security Administration that includes name, social security number, date of birth, and date of death, cancer registrars are able to complete follow-up information with dates of death that they may not have had access to.

As a data analyst, you need to be sure that you are using valid, reliable data. An awareness of the issues involved in data scrubbing is important before you invest your time in data analysis. Once your data are clean, you can move on to the concept of data mapping.

> **Data constraints** Rules that limit the type of data that can be entered into a field.

> **TAKE AWAY**
>
> The data dictionary establishes data constraints that control how data items are collected, ensuring data quality.

> **Data harmonization** The process of formatting all data items in a similar manner.

> **Data enhancement** The activity of adding information by checking against a validated database.

EXERCISE 9-2
Data Scrubbing

1. The field for Social Security number accepts only XXX-XX-XXXX and not, for example, XXXXXXXXX. What type of data constraint is this?

2. A field asks for patient Social Security number, regardless of format. What type of data constraint is this?

3. Some of the physicians are recording patient insurance by abbreviation, and some are using a number to represent the type of insurance. What type of data constraint is this?

4. You notice that some of the discharge dates are for 2024. What type of data constraint is this?

5. One of your physicians is using a coded set for gender that is M (male), F (female), and U (unknown). What type of data constraint is this?

6. You notice that the patient's medical record numbers are missing in your print out. What type of data constraint is this?

DATA MAPPING

EHR Electronic health record.

Data mapping The process of matching elements between distinct data sets.

Source In data mapping, the original data set mapped to the target.

Target In data mapping, the data set to which the source is mapped.

Not all data are collected with the same instrument, same database rules, EHR program, or with the same classification systems. Fortunately, this does not always inhibit an analyst from comparing different data sets. The process of matching elements between distinct data sets is called **data mapping**. It involves figuring out which items are similar (called *equivalence* or *synonymy*), which items are a part of a larger group, and which have no equal—those which are unique to the set.

You may be familiar with *general equivalence mappings (GEMs)*, used to translate ICD-9-CM codes to ICD-10-CM/PCS codes and vice versa. Using GEMs to trend data with ICD-10-CM required an analysis to determine the relationships between each of the ICD-9 codes and their ICD-10 equivalents. This is one of the uses of mapping. Mapping is also useful when there is a software change that uses different names or formats for patient information. A map is necessary to allow the information from one database to be integrated and added to the new one.

The data set that the information is mapped *from* is called the **source**. The data set that the information is mapped *to* is called the **target** (Fig. 9-2). A physician's practice might want to compare the diagnoses treated by their practitioners before and after they joined the practice. Because the information was recorded by different EHR systems, it will be necessary to map the data fields representing the diagnoses to the practice's current EHR system. The former data fields are the sources, while the current data fields in the practice's EHR system are the targets.

TAKE AWAY

Data mapping allows databases to be compared or combined, even if the data items in each database have been collected and recorded in different formats.

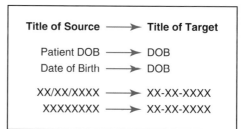

Figure 9-2 An example of data mapping.

BRIEF CASE

MAPPING DATA

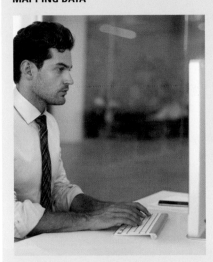

The previous EHR system used all ICD-9-CM codes, but the study Hector is working on would go well into years that are covered by ICD-10-CM/PCS codes. The vendor for the system had done the mapping, but Hector needs to check some of the codes. His infectious disease department wants to make sure that their caseload will be able to be trended with the new ICD-10-CM codes. One of their specific requests was the Ebola virus.

Hector sets up a table to include all of the diagnoses that needed to be mapped between ICD-9-CM and ICD-10-CM for the infectious diseases requested by his physicians. He knows that he will need to keep an eye on any changes that came from CMS (Centers for Medicare and Medicaid Services) in the future, but for now, he has a start on knowing which codes are assigned to the diagnoses in question.

CMS Centers for medicare and medicaid services.

Some are already in ICD-10-CM, and she needs to find the ICD-9-CM code, while others are only in ICD-9-CM with no ICD-10-CM equivalent. She reviews the following table for errors and needs to correct any found. Use http://www.icd9data.com/or another resource of your choice to map the missing codes.

DISEASE/DISORDER	ICD-9-CM	ICD-10-CM
Rubella, NOS	056.9	
Rubeola, NOS	055.9	
Mumps, without complication		B26.9
Tuberculosis of lung, infiltrative, unspecified		A15.0
Syphilis, unspecified	097.9	
Rabies, unspecified		A82.9
Varicella, NOS		B01.9
Poliomyelitis, acute paralytic, unspecified	045.1	
Diphtheria, unspecified	032.9	
Pertussis, unspecified	033.9	
Ebola virus disease		A98.4

The rules that are used in the mapping process are referred to as **heuristics**. For example, if the individual's marital status is to be categorized as M for married, S for single, D for divorced, and W for widowed, then a different system using numbers for each (for example, 1 for single) will need to be mapped to the current system's categorization. The heuristic would use the source of 1 for single and map it to S whenever that category is encountered in the data set. Another way to analyze the data is categorize all those who are single together, and a second category can be "not single." This may improve interpretation of the data.

Heuristics The rules governing how one set of data is mapped to another.

Mapping should be considered a work in progress, as one must continually keep the mapping updated. Changes (such as code changes) must be added to the map on a routine basis to keep the integrity of the data intact. All maps need to be dated as of their last maintenance activity.

EXERCISE 9-3
Data Mapping

1. What is the term that describes the database that the case is mapped from?

2. What is the term that describes the rules that are used for mapping?

3. Another term for synonymy, this describes the equal relationship between items that are being mapped.

4. Database X is mapped to Database Y. In this example, Database Y is the _____.

REVIEW QUESTIONS

1. The proposed 2016 database for comparing lengths of stay for the surgical unit includes a field for the patient diagnosis recorded with ICD-9-CM. This is an example of an issue with which type of data quality? _____.

2. Physician A has recorded patient weights in pounds, while physician B has all of the weights in kilograms. This is an issue of data _____.

3. Several patients have not stated their religious preference. This is an issue of data _____.

4. Yesterday, while reviewing the addresses of the client list, Diane noticed that there were problems with how the practice was recording route numbers. Some were recorded as the abbreviation "Rt" and some as "Rte," and others were spelled out completely. She changed all of the abbreviations to the full spelling of route. What kind of data scrubbing did she do?

5. Zip codes that start with a capital O instead of a zero are examples of a lack of _____.

6. Using rules that changed each zip code to nine digits and every date of birth to two-digit month, two-digit day, and four-digit year are examples of what?

7. A patient's medical record number appears in the patient's lab and imaging reports. This is an example of a _____.

8. Brandy realized that she needed to set a _____ constraint that prevents the admission date from being after the discharge date.

9. Andrea used an ICD-10-CM code when she mapped it to the ICD-9-CM code. Is the ICD-9-CM code the source or the target?

10. Dr. Winston had one of the first EHR systems in his city. When he joined the hospital practice, the way that insurance was abbreviated and categorized was different. Mapping from the doctor's old system to the hospital system used what type of constraint?

11. Ida Johnson, DOB 4/15/1956, appeared to be the same as Ida R. Johnson, DOB 4/15/1956, and Ida Ruth Johnson, DOB 4/15/1956. Checking to be sure that this patient is the same ensures _____.

PREDICTING DATA

CHAPTER OUTLINE

KEY TERMS

alternate hypothesis
central limit theorem (CLT)
confidence intervals
confidence level
correlation
inferential statistics
non-probability sampling

null hypothesis
p values
population
probability
probability sampling
random sampling
sample

sampling bias
sampling error
significance
standard error (SE)
type I error
type II error

LEARNING OBJECTIVES

At the conclusion of this chapter, you should be able to do the following:

1. Differentiate between descriptive and inferential statistics.
2. Explain the importance of random sampling in inferential statistics.
3. Define confidence intervals and levels.
4. Define significance.
5. Calculate standard error.
6. Define hypothesis testing.
7. Define and identify type I and type II errors.

INTRODUCTION

Earlier chapters explained how to describe data both numerically and graphically, along with how to have clean, coordinated data. They covered a variety of statistics that can be used to examine a data set: calculations that included volume, averages, and variance. Those calculations are illustrated in a number of different tables, charts, and graphs.

Statistics, however, are not only descriptive but also predictive. Where descriptive statistics help us organize and describe data collected from a specified population, **inferential statistics** allow us to make generalizations about that population from a sample. With inferential statistics, we can make assumptions about what our *sample* data is telling us about our *population.*

- *Is the length of stay longer for an open or laparoscopic type of surgery?*
- *Is productivity the same for both remote and in-house coders?*
- *Which nursing shift has the greatest number of medical errors?*

Because of the power of inferential statistics to make predictions about entire populations, we can add to the body of knowledge with what we know to be true about whatever we have examined. The most powerful example of this is the prospective payment system (PPS). Using data from patient hospital stays, the government is able to predict what the cost and length of stay (LOS) will be for most patients with similar diagnoses and procedures.

> **Inferential statistics** The study of using mathematical models to predict future events.

> **LOS** Length of stay.

> **TAKE AWAY** ●·········
>
> Data analysis can be used to not only describe the data that we already have in our facilities but predict the results of future events.

BRIEF CASE

PREDICTING THE FUTURE

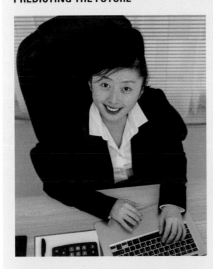

As a Data Systems Analyst for the Diamonte Health system, Aiko performs data set construction, management, and the analysis and presentation of information for the entire enterprise, consisting of hospitals and physician practices. She thinks there might be a connection between the use of the provider's patient portal—the Website where patients can make appointments, view lab results, request prescription refills, and gain other access to their personal health information—and a patient's health literacy, or how much they understand health information and available services.

Aiko is also providing support for one of the physicians on the teaching staff at her hospital system. The physician has recently noticed that several pairs of identical twins in his practice have diabetes. He wonders if there is any connection between the A1c levels of these identical twins. While most of her daily tasks have to do with providing descriptive statistics, today Aiko will be involved with its cousin, inferential statistics. She is going to help determine if there is a statistical relationship between the A1c levels of identical twins that this particular physician is treating and the incidence of type I diabetes. Using what she knows, she is going to try to *predict* what will happen in the future for other identical twins with diabetes.

POPULATIONS AND SAMPLES

Inferential statistics is a branch of mathematics that allows us to make predictions about an entire population from sample data. A **population** is a grouping that includes every actual or potential element, item, or individual under study. For example, if a data

> **Population** An entire group; every actual or potential element, item, or individual under study.

Sample A smaller group within a population.

Sampling error The possibility that the mean of the sample is different from the mean of the population, and therefore not representative of the entire population.

Significance A measure of the reliability of an observed effect.

Sampling bias A distortion of the true nature of the population, caused by non-random sampling.

Probability sampling A sample selection method that seeks to avoid bias by choosing a random selection.

analyst is asked to examine the relationship between the incidence of pressure ulcers and LOS, the population would have to include all patients who had ever had a pressure ulcer. Because the numbers would be prohibitive to study, subsets of a population, or **samples**, are used. The sample data is used to tell you what you could expect if you measured every last one of the entire population. They are predictive in two senses: (1) from the sample to the population and (2) from the sample to the future for similar populations.

It is important that the sample selected from the population retain the essential characteristics of the population. Because the samples are only a part of the population they are drawn from, there is a varying degree of uncertainty about these predictions.

Sampling error is the concept that whenever we draw a sample, there is an inherent possibility that our sample (although not biased) does not reflect the characteristics of the entire population, and hence, our sampling means can be different from the population mean. We will use the concept of sampling error later in the chapter to help us determine how likely our sampling results have given us a reliable result.

Statistical **significance** is a measure of *how likely* it is that the results were simply by chance, as opposed to being a statistical association. For example, is there a relationship, an association, between the incidence of pressure ulcers and a patient's LOS? Essentially, significance tells us how reliable our results are. This measure is a statistical calculation that estimates the probability that an association is present between the variables under study.

To establish a statistically significant relationship, analysts must choose an appropriate sampling method. Sampling methods can be divided into two general categories: *probability sampling* and *non-probability sampling*. Sometimes, the conclusions we draw from a sample are false because the sample is not a truly random selection of the population. **Sampling bias** is a distortion of the true nature of the population; it is the result of non-random sampling and causes some members of the population to have a lesser chance of being chosen for the sample than others. Say, for example, a political candidate used a smartphone app to gather voters' opinions on the issues. The results gathered from such a survey would be biased because smartphone users are not representative of the entire population of voters. **Probability samples** are those that seek to avoid bias by choosing a random selection of patients for their study. Table 10-1 lists various methods of probability sampling and gives examples of each method.

TABLE 10-1

SAMPLING METHODS

METHOD	DEFINITION	EXAMPLE
Probability Sampling		
Cluster sample	Divides a population into groups, a number of those groups are randomly selected, and then each member of those groups is then studied.	An analyst wants to know how long inpatient coders stay with the same employer. All the inpatient coders in the region are divided into groups by hospital, and 10 hospitals are selected at random. Researchers interview all the inpatient coders at each of the 10 hospitals.
Simple random sample	Each member of the population has the same chance of being selected as any other member.	A random number table is used to choose 100 patients who were treated in the last month for a satisfaction survey using their medical record numbers.

Continued

TABLE 10-1—cont'd

METHOD	DEFINITION	EXAMPLE
Systematic random sample	The choice of element is the *n*th number of a population.	The hospital system had 2000 births last year, and the administrator wants to survey the mothers to assess the feasibility of a midwifery suite. A sample of those patients can be obtained by choosing every 25th patient after randomly choosing the first patient.
Stratified random sample	Divides the population into strata, or groups of similar patients (by age, sex, surgical service, disposition), and a set number of members within each strata is studied.	Patients are being studied for their satisfaction within a physician practice. Patients are grouped by the variables of age, sex, insurance type, and physician. The strata are then used for a random selection of patients to ensure an even selection for the variables in question.

Non-Probability Sampling

METHOD	DEFINITION	EXAMPLE
Convenience sample	Used to easily (and inexpensively) approximate results without the time and expense of a probability sample.	A group of patients volunteer for a study; a day's worth of test results are examined; the opinions of the physicians of the nearest clinic are gathered.
Judgment sample	Relies entirely on the common sense of the researcher doing the study; may be an extension of convenience sampling.	Researchers looking for an association between alcohol/drug abuse and the incidence of certain sexually transmitted diseases obtain a sample of health records from a clinic that has a staff that is willing to participate by abstracting the required data elements.
Quota sample	Aims to attain a sample that has similar proportions to the general population. The sample is divided into groups that represent the variables that are being examined. The proportions of these groups are noted, and then the subjects are chosen according to that proportion.	Researchers want to study of levels of severity of illness by age and sex. The population is first divided into the number of levels of severity under study, then each of them by age and sex. The final sample is chosen by applying the proportions of each to the subgroups.
Snowball sample	The sample is chosen through the use of referrals from any individuals who are identified; used when the subject under study is difficult to find (rare diseases or conditions, for example).	Patients with Marfan syndrome, a rare genetic disorder affecting the connective tissue of the body, contact other patients who have the same condition and ask them to participate.

For some studies, however, the sample is not random, and no effort is made to ensure a random sample. Obtaining a random sample of a population can be difficult, after all, and researchers are frequently constrained by time and costs. This is called **non-probability sampling**, and while it can provide meaningful results, there is no mathematical calculation that can tell the analysts if they have represented the population well. If you have ever seen a news segment on television where the reporter stops people on a city street to ask their opinion on current events, you have seen non-probability sampling in action. Various methods of non-probability sampling are also listed in Table 10-1.

Non-probability sampling A sample selection method that does not seek to avoid bias and in which the selection is not done randomly.

BRIEF CASE

SELECTING A SAMPLE

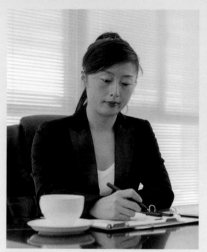

Aiko wants to ask patients whether they have ever logged onto the provider's patient portal, and if so, how often. She would also like to know what types of patient portal services they use. A more detailed survey will be given later to judge each patient's understanding of their health and the types of services offered to them, but first, she needs to find some patients to include in the sample. Aiko brainstorms the following sampling methods. Match each example with the name of the method.

_____ 1. Every fifth patient will be given a survey card at the patient checkout.	A. Cluster sample
_____ 2. All patients whose Social Security number ends in the number 3 will be mailed a survey.	B. Convenience sample
_____ 3. All patients who visited the physician practice on Wednesday are given a survey.	C. Systematic random sample
_____ 4. Patients are divided into groups by age range and gender. Ten individuals are chosen from each group by drawing names out of a hat.	D. Stratified random sample

PROBABILITY

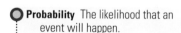

Probability The likelihood that an event will happen.

At the heart of inferential statistics is the concept of **probability**, the likelihood that an event will happen. Every day we use probability when we check the weather forecast for the risk of rain, listen to the news about the possible outcome of an election, or consider the chance of winning a jackpot lottery. As many of our other concepts in statistics, this is expressed as a number, often a percentage, and the symbol used is a p. Here are some common examples of probabilities:

- On Thursday, there is a 10% chance of rain.
- The latest polls show Smith will get 53% of the vote, with a standard error of ± 2.
- Officials calculate each ticket sold has a 1 in 60 million chance of winning the lottery.

The reason why all of this happens is based on the normal distribution. If you think back to our coverage of standard deviation in Chapter 2, you might remember that these normal curves are based on standard deviations from the mean, represented by the Greek letter sigma (σ), where one σ comprises 68% of the observations, two σ 95%, and three σ 99%. In the bell curve, the graphical representation of the results of data collection, the greatest number of responses will be gathered around the average response (Figure 10-1).

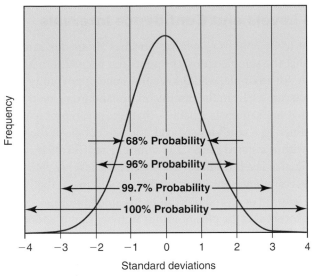

Figure 10-1 A bell curve.

Central Limit Theorem (CLT)

With a large enough sample (usually 30 or greater), the sample means will be normally distributed even if the scores themselves are not. This is called the **central limit theorem (CLT)**, and it is what allows us to use sampling to make our predictions, instead of examining each and every member of a population. We can use the CLT concept to determine if our data is (or is not) within the limits of a standardized normal distribution to test hypotheses about the data. It allows us to standardize our observations so that we can compare them.

> **Central limit theorem (CLT)** The mathematical rule stating that the observations of a sample will be distributed normally if the sample is large enough.

Standard Error

A calculation that is necessary to meaningfully compare our observations is called standard error. Standard error is a measure of how sampling error affects your results. While standard deviation measures how different the scores are in the population being measured, **standard error (SE)** measures the difference between the *means of samples* of that population. Standard error is actually a standard deviation of the sample mean. If the standard error of those means is large, then the sample means are very different from each other. If the standard error of the means is small, then it follows that they are very similar to each other. When choosing your sample size, you can be sure that the larger your sample size, the smaller your standard error. Think about it this way: the sample mean would be the same as the population mean if you "sampled" every single item in the population.

> **Standard error (SE)** The difference between the means of samples of a population.

The formula for standard error is the standard deviation divided by the square root of the size of the sample. For example, if the sample of our population of 100 patients with a mean age of 22 has a standard deviation of 12 and our sample size is 9, the standard error is 12 divided by 3 (the square root of 9), or 4. This would mean that you can expect that the mean of your sample lies within one standard deviation of your mean ± 4 (so between $22 - 4$ and $22 + 4$). Another way of saying this is that you have about a 68% chance of your sample mean being within that range because 68% represents one standard deviation, or the chance of being correct two out of three times.

Confidence Levels and Confidence Intervals

Because we want to be able to generalize findings about our sample, we need to be *reasonably sure* that the sample truly represents our population. That means that each and every patient, for example, would have the same opportunity of being chosen for the sample. As you can see from the discussion of standard error, the larger our sample, the more likely that our sample is reliable—that is to say, repeatable. "Reasonably sure" in statistics is defined as a **confidence level,** the percentage of the population that will yield an answer within a stated range. The symbol *p* represents probability and is associated with confidence levels. Usually, the confidence level is 95% (*p* = 0.95), although sometimes a 99% confidence level is used. That would mean that 95% (or 99%) of the time, you can be assured of a similar result to the study finding.

A **confidence interval** is the plus or minus number that is added to (and subtracted from) the result that you have calculated and is derived from your standard error calculation. The most familiar use of this is during an election. You may have heard of a survey resulting in "53% of the people studied will vote for a given candidate with a margin of error of ± 2 percentage points." The confidence interval is the ± 2%. If the confidence level is 95%, it means that there is a 95% chance that 51% to 55% of the population will vote for that particular candidate.

To determine a confidence interval, there are three considerations: *sample size, population size,* and *percentage that chooses the particular result.* First, consider the size of the sample. A larger sample would most likely yield a result more reflective of the total population. Because of that, the larger the sample, the smaller the confidence interval will be. If your population is small and your sample is large, you can be more confident that your result is reliable. If 100 people ordered the soup in the cafeteria and you surveyed 80 of them, you could be confident in your results. However, if your population is very large and your sample is small, the likelihood of a reliable result is much smaller. Finally, if 9800 of 10,000 patients discharged last year, or 98% of your patients (the population sampled), say that they are "very satisfied" with the service they received at your hospital, you can be very sure that reporting a sample of that result—as the most frequent response—is reliable.

For example, let us say a physician practice has undergone an analysis of their adolescent BMIs to explore the possibility of a new program to deal with teenage obesity. Three samples of varying size were drawn to calculate standard error to be used in determining confidence levels and intervals. As you can see from our illustration below, the larger the sample size, the lower the standard error. Using 95% confidence levels, sample 1 would be 27 ± 2 for a range of 23 to 31 (remember to double the SE for each SD; here we have two), and in sample 3, the range would be 30 ± 0.5 or 29–31. You can see how increasing the sample size narrows the range and allows us to make conclusions that we can be much surer of.

> **Confidence level** The percentage of the population that will yield an answer within a stated range.

> ## MATH REVIEW
>
> Do you notice the connection to 2 standard deviations from the mean? It describes a much more "confident" result than our 1 standard deviation of 68%.

	Sample 1	Sample 2	Sample 3
Mean:	27	31	30
SD, *s*:	6	4	3
Sample Size, *n*:	9	16	36
Sqrt(*n*):	3	4	6
SE = *s*/sqrt of *n*:	6/3 = 2.0	4/4 = 1.0	3/6 = 0.5

Testing to see if your findings are significant requires setting up a hypothesis and statistically determining whether your results meet your requirements for being "reasonably sure." We will introduce the methods and some of the calculations for hypothesis testing in the next section.

EXERCISE 10-1
Samples, Populations, and Probability

1. Inferential statistics are dependent on the concept of _____, the likelihood that an event will happen.

2. Convenience, judgment, and quota sampling are all examples of what type of sampling technique?

3. What is a subset or part of a population under study?

4. What type of sampling category uses a random selection of a population?

5. What type of sample would you be using if you gave surveys to the first 50 patients who arrived for appointments at your outpatient clinic?

6. If you decide to examine every seventh medical record for a particular type of procedure, what type of sampling method are you using?

7. One of your medical services asks that you sample 50 patients for each physician in regard to their satisfaction with their care. What type of sampling method are you using?

8. What percentage of observations will be $\pm 1 \sigma$ outside of the mean in a normal distribution?

9. In a class of 251 students, the sample of 25 students had a mean score of 77. The standard deviation of the sample mean is 7. What is the confidence level at 95%?

HYPOTHESIS TESTING

Inferential statistics can help you use the concepts of probability and confidence levels to determine if you have found a new bit of "truth." Most studies look for either differences or associations between groups of data. For example, you might think that men have a longer LOS than the average for a specified diagnosis, or that there is a difference in the average age for a given diagnosis, or that by taking a particular drug, there is a drop in blood pressure. How could you test that? There is a logical sequence to figuring out if your explanation for your data, your hypothesis, is true or not.

1. **State the null hypothesis.** To begin, you need to test your hypothesis by stating what is called a **null hypothesis**: a statement of no difference between the men's LOS and the average LOS of a given diagnosis-related group (DRG), or between the average case mix of one doctor and another. The symbol for the null hypothesis is H_0. Your hypothesis, expecting a difference between the two, is referred to as the **alternative hypothesis**, and the symbol is H_1. The alternative hypothesis will be accepted if the null hypothesis is rejected.

Stat Tip

An easy way to remember is that null is from the Latin meaning "not any" or "none." Notice that the subscript is also a zero. Both of those serve to remind you that the null hypothesis claims there is **no** difference between the variables being examined.

TAKE AWAY

Hypothesis testing is the statistical method of determining how likely a future event can be or how likely your sample represents the entire population.

○ **Null hypothesis** A statement that there is no relationship between the specified populations.

○ **LOS** Length of stay.

○ **Diagnosis-related group** A health care description of statistically similar categories of diagnoses.

○ **Alternative hypothesis** The relationship between two populations expected by a data analyst.

$H_0 = $ null hypothesis $H_1 = $ alternative hypothesis

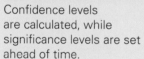
ALOS Average length of stay.

For example, let us say we suspect men have a greater ALOS than the ALOS for a certain diagnosis for all patients of a given DRG at your hospital. The null hypothesis is that there is no difference between the ALOS and the general population of patients. Expressed as a formula, we would say that $H_0: \mu_1 = \mu_2$, where the ALOS for men $= \mu_1$ and the ALOS for the population $= \mu_2$. If there is no difference (they are the same), then the result of subtraction would be 0. The alternative hypothesis is that there **is** a difference between the average LOS for men and the population $(\mu_1 > \mu_2)$. Notice that the alternative does not determine *how* they are different, it just tests that there is a detectable difference.

2. Next, you need to **set up a significance level.** Significance is a measure of how reliable the result is. It tells you how sure you can be that resampling would yield a similar result. The levels are usually 0.05 (most commonly) or 0.01. Another way of looking at these numbers is that 0.05 and 0.01 means 95% and 99% of the time, respectively, like in our last example in the probability section. For example, a significance level of 0.02 means that if you gathered an entirely new sample, you would get the same result 98% of the time. The symbol for the chosen significance level is α, as in $\alpha = 0.05$. Results are then stated as the study "being significant at the 0.05 (or 0.01) level."

3. **Calculate.** Once a significance level is set, it is time to go ahead and calculate whatever it is that you are testing.

4. **Find the *p* value.** Using your results, you next need to calculate the probability of obtaining the same findings (a *p* value) and compare it to the significance level that you had previously set. The *p* **value** tells you the chance that you calculate a statistic different from the one that you have stated in your null hypothesis.

5. **Accept or reject the null.** *If the probability (p value) is less than or equal to the significance level that you have selected*, then the null hypothesis is rejected. If the probability is greater than the significance level you have set, the null is not rejected and your findings are considered to be "statistically significant."

Sometimes significance can be confused with *p* values and confidence levels. Significance is the alpha level that is the *predetermined* measure you are using to determine if you accept or reject your null hypothesis. You would want to have a very small significance level in a drug study to show the efficacy of its effect, where you might not be quite as concerned with a study of how likely patients are to respond to reminders for upcoming appointments. *P* values are the chance that your sample falls within that level: they are the probability of your particular calculated result occurring.

Another way of analyzing data to test a hypothesis is to look for an association between two variables. For example, the amount of time spent studying for an exam is usually related to the results on that exam. The number of hours after a meal is related to the perception of hunger by an individual. To determine if a statistical relationship exists, the variables need to be on similar scales. For example, if you want to compare those hours of study with the results on an exam, you would need to convert each of those measures (hours and exam grades) into standard (z) scores, so that they can be analyzed. Standard (z) scores are determined by subtracting the mean from each score and dividing it by the standard deviation.

$$Z = \frac{x - \text{mean of } x}{\text{SD}}$$

If the scores are on the same scale, the conversion to z scores is not necessary.

The *Pearson product-moment correlation coefficient* is used with ordinal and ratio level data. The *Spearman rank-order correlation coefficient* is used only with ordinal scales, with nominal scales not being an issue because they can not be ordered (red/blue/green, male/female). The symbol for correlation is ϱ (rho) and the values of

---

TAKE AWAY •·········

Significance levels are set to choose the degree of likelihood *ahead of testing*. They are used with the testing to figure out how likely the results determined can be replicated.

---

p value The probability of mistakenly rejecting the null hypothesis when it is in fact true.

TAKE AWAY •·········

Confidence levels are calculated, while significance levels are set ahead of time.

TAKE AWAY •·········

The null hypothesis states there is no difference between the data and the mean observations (or correlation levels), while the alternate hypothesis (the one that the researcher is hoping to prove) states that there *is* a significant difference.

association are from a positive to a negative (+1.00 to −1.00). A correlation of +1.00 would mean that every time a patient has a high score on one variable, they have an analogous high score on the related variable. A −1.00 correlation would mean that every time a patient has a high score on one variable, they have an analogous low value on the opposite variable. A correlation of 0.0 would mean that there is no correlation between the two variables.

The formula for the Pearson correlation coefficient is $P = \Sigma \dfrac{(Zx \times Zy)}{N}$, where N is the number of paired observations.

TESTING A HYPOTHESIS

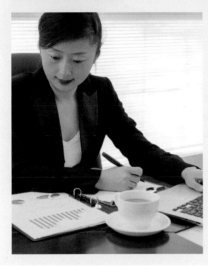

Aiko has determined her sample of patients from the enterprise database. She has results on 12 paired twins with their Alc levels and is ready to test to see if there is any relationship between the twins' Alc readings. Her null hypothesis is that there is no relationship between the twins' readings. She determines that there is a 0.7 correlation between the pairs of twins that is significant at the 0.05 level.

Does she accept or reject the null hypothesis for this study?
What type of correlation would this be: positive, negative, or no correlation?

Type I and Type II Errors

Proving your hypothesis can be hazardous. Once you have written your null and alternative hypotheses, your significance levels, and the calculation of your *p* values, you need to confront the possibility of two types of errors that may occur and why.

A **type I error** is when you reject a null hypothesis when it is really true. A **type II error** is the opposite, which is accepting the null hypothesis when it is false. (See Figure 10-2). Here are some examples:

- Type I error: Researchers claim there is a difference in survival times between patients who are treated with a particular drug and those who were given a placebo—when there really is not. Patients who were given the drug lived for the same length of time as those who received the placebo. This is also called a *false positive*.
- Type II error: Researchers claim there is no difference in the survival time between patients who are treated with a particular drug and those who were given a placebo—when there actually is. The patients who took the drug lived an average of 6 months longer than those who were given the placebo. This is also called a *false negative*.

The chance of making a type I error is tied to the level of significance that is chosen. Remember that statistical significance is a measure of the percentage of times you can repeat the result with a new sample. If your significance level is 0.05, then you expect to repeat your result 95% of the time. You expect a result that proves the null hypothesis 5% of the time, or 1 in 20 times, and at a significance of 0.05; you accept that result. If the consequences of a type I error are serious or expensive, then a very small significance level is appropriate. Choosing a level that is too high or too low can lead to both of these types of errors. Figure 10-3 summarizes type I and type II errors.

Type I error The rejection of the null hypothesis when it is actually true.

Type II error The acceptance of the null hypothesis when it is actually false.

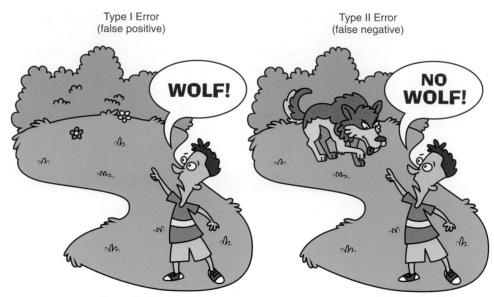

Figure 10-2 The difference between type I and type II errors.

Decision (based on sample)	Truth (for population studied)	
	Null Hypothesis True	Null Hypothesis False
Reject Null Hypothesis	Type I Error	Correct Decision
Fail to reject Null Hypothesis	Correct Decision	Type II Error

A

Verdict	Truth	
	Not Guilty	Guilty
Guilty	Type I Error Innocent person goes to jail (and may be guilty person goes free)	Correct Decision
Not Guilty	Correct Decision	Type II Error Guilty person goes free

B

Decision	Truth	
	Not Effective	Effective
Effective	Type I Error Drug that does not work is passed on as effective.	Correct Decision
Not Effective	Correct Decision	Type II Error Effective drug is considered ineffective and is never developed.

C

Figure 10-3 Summary and Examples of Type I and Type II Errors. A, Table showing summary of decision and error types. **B,** The concept of a jury trial and verdicts is often used to clarify the difference between type I and type II errors. **C,** An example based on the acceptance or rejection of a pharmaceutical.

TAKE AWAY ●·····························

A type I error stems from the chance (your significance level, for example, 0.05) of making a wrong decision when your null hypothesis is true. A type II error means coming to the wrong conclusion when your null hypothesis is false. Just remember that these errors are based on the significance level that is set ahead of time, and setting a significance level too high (or too low) can alter your results.

EXERCISE 10-2

Hypothesis Testing

1. The research hypothesis that assumes no difference between the findings is called the _____ hypothesis.

2. Rejecting the null hypothesis when it is actually true is what type of error?

3. The opposite of the null hypothesis is the _____ hypothesis.

4. Accepting the null hypothesis when it is actually not true is which type of error? _____

5. The likelihood of a false result is referred to as statistical _____.

REVIEW QUESTIONS

1. What type of statistics helps us organize and describe data collected from a specified population?

2. What type of statistics helps us make assumptions about the sample data?

3. What term describes the likelihood that an event will happen?

4. What term describes the standard deviation of the sample means?

5. What is the name of the concept that allows us to generalize our findings to the population from a sample of 30 or greater?

6. What is the term for a grouping that includes every actual or potential element under study?

7. What is the term for the result of non-random sampling that causes some members of the population to have a lesser chance of being chosen for the sample than others?

8. What type of sampling category does not seek to avoid sampling bias?

9. Researchers studying health care insurance coverage in the city isolated people by city blocks. They then randomly chose eight blocks and surveyed every household on those eight blocks. What type of sampling method did they use?

10. A _____ sample is one in which each member of the population has the same chance of being selected as any other member.

11. Choosing every fifth member of a population is an example of a _____ random sample.

12. A _____ random sample divides the population into groups of similar patients and then studies the patients within that group.

13. Using the entire group of patients who appeared at a clinic on one day of the week for your study is an example of a _____ sample.

14. A researcher wants to study how fatigued women who have lupus feel at certain stages of their menstrual cycle. The researcher gathers her sample by selecting only patients who have lupus. What type of sampling is this?

15. Enrollment at the university is 55% female, 45% male, 60% African-American, 40% white or Caucasian, 15% Hispanic or Latino, and 5% Asian or Pacific Islander. When studying the amount of sleep students get each night, the graduate student is careful to ensure the sample represents these demographic characteristics. What type of sampling is this?

16. Using referrals from individuals with an unusual condition is an example of _____ sampling.

17. Explain the difference between the confidence level and the significance level.

18. The A1c readings of 81 patients were taken at a practice before their treatment. The population of all the patients is 742. The sample mean is 6.3, and the standard deviation of the mean is 0.9. What is the standard error, confidence level at 99%, and confidence interval?

19. What is the first step of hypothesis testing?

20. Marketers report that 60% of individuals ages 18–25 do not have a landline phone in their primary residence, +/– 3%. The plus or minus added to the result is called the _____.

21. A statement of no difference between variables is considered a _____ hypothesis.

22. Mistakenly concluding that a difference exists when it does not is considered which type of error?

23. Concluding that there is no difference between variables when one exists is considered which type of error?

24. The new data analyst was given a task to choose a group of patients from one of the cardiology practices for a survey to determine how the patients made the choice of their physician. She was asked to include sex, age, zip code, and insurance type. The intent of the study was to conclude whether any of the factors studied were related to the choice of a particular physician.

    a. What type of statistics will be used to make conclusions about the findings?
    b. The group of all patients treated by the practice is referred to as a _____?
    c. Should she use a probability or non-probability sample?
    d. What type of sampling technique should she use?
    e. If one of the hypotheses is stated as "There is no difference between the sex of the patient and their choice of physician" that would represent which type of hypothesis?

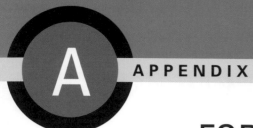

APPENDIX

FORMULA QUICK REFERENCE

Calculating Occupancy

$$\frac{\text{Total inpatient service days}}{\text{Total inpatient bed count days}} \times 100 = \% \text{ Occupancy}$$

Calculating a Basic Rate

$$\frac{\text{Number of times something occurred in a time period}}{\text{Number of times it could have occurred in the same time period}} \times 100$$

Calculating an HAI Rate

$$\frac{\text{Total number of infections after 48 (or 72 hours) of hospitalization for a period}}{\text{Total number of discharges (including deaths) for a period}} \times 100$$

Calculating an Infection Rate

$$\frac{\text{Total number of infections in a given month}}{\text{Total number of patients discharged for the same month}} \times 100$$

Calculating a Postoperative Infection Rate

$$\frac{\text{Total number of postoperative infections}}{\text{Total number of clean surgical procedures}} \times 100$$

Calculating Ventilator-Associated Pneumonia in Discharged Patients

$$\frac{\text{Patients with VAP for a time period}}{\text{Discharged patients who were on a mechanical ventilator for a time period}} \times 100$$

Calculating Ventilator Usage

$$\frac{\text{Patients on mechanical ventilators for a time period}}{\text{Patients discharged for a time period}} \times 100$$

Calculating Infection Rate Compared to Days on Ventilator

$$\frac{\text{Patients with VAP for a time period}}{\text{Ventilator days for a time period}} \times 100$$

Calculating Consultation Rates Using Total Number of Patients Seen

$$\frac{\text{Total number of patients seen by a consultant}}{\text{Total number of discharges (including deaths)}} \times 100$$

Calculating Consultation Rates Using Total Number of Consultations

$$\frac{\text{Total number of consultations (reports) provided}}{\text{Total number of discharges (including deaths)}} \times 100$$

Calculating the Fetal Death Rate

$$\frac{\text{Total number of fetal deaths for a period}}{\text{Total number of births + fetal deaths for this period}} \times 100$$

Calculating Cesarean Section Rates

$$\frac{\text{Total number of Cesarean sections for a period}}{\text{Total number of deliveries (live or dead) for this period}} \times 100$$

Calculating VBAC Rates

$$\frac{\text{Total number vaginal deliveries among women who had prior Cesarean sections}}{\text{Total number of Cesarean section births among women who had prior Cesarean sections}} \times 100$$

✏ Calculating Maternal Mortality Rates

$$\frac{\text{Total number of maternal deaths for a period}}{\text{Total number of discharges from the OB wards (including deaths) for this period}} \times 100$$

✏ Calculating Newborn Mortality Rates

$$\frac{\text{Total number of newborn deaths for a period}}{\text{Total number of newborn discharges (including deaths) for this period}} \times 100$$

✏ Calculating Neonatal Mortality Rates

$$\frac{\text{Total number of neonatal deaths for a period}}{\text{Total number of neonatal discharges (including deaths) for this period}} \times 100$$

✏ Calculating Gross Mortality Rates

$$\frac{\text{Total number of inpatient deaths}}{\text{Total number of discharges (including deaths)}} \times 100$$

✏ Calculating Net Mortality Rates

$$\frac{\text{Total number of inpatient deaths (including newborns)} - \text{deaths} < 48 \text{ hours after admission}}{\text{Total number of discharges (including newborns)} - \text{deaths} < 48 \text{ hours after admission}} \times 100$$

✏ Calculating Postoperative Mortality Rates

$$\frac{\text{Total surgical deaths within 10 days postop}}{\text{Total surgical patients}} \times 100$$

✏ Calculating Anesthesia Death Rates

$$\frac{\text{Total deaths due to anesthesia}}{\text{Total number of times anesthesia was administered}} \times 100,000$$

Calculating Gross Autopsy Rates

$$\frac{\text{Total number of autopsies performed on inpatients for a period}}{\text{Total number of inpatient deaths for this period}} \times 100$$

Calculating Net Autopsy Rates

$$\frac{\text{Total number of autopsies performed on inpatients for a period}}{\text{Total number of IP deaths-those bodies removed by MEs for this period}} \times 100$$

Calculating Adjusted (Hospital) Autopsy Rates

$$\frac{\begin{array}{c}\text{Total number of autopsies performed on inpatients} \\ \text{+ autopsies on former patients} \\ \text{- bodies removed by the ME for a period}\end{array}}{\begin{array}{c}\text{Total number of IP deaths} \\ \text{+ bodies of former patients available for autopsy} \\ \text{- those bodies removed by MEs for this period}\end{array}} \times 100$$

Calculating Fetal Death Autopsy Rates

$$\frac{\text{Total number of autopsies performed on fetal deaths for a period}}{\text{Total number of fetal deaths for this period}} \times 100$$

Calculating Pediatric Autopsy Rates

Note: you will need to consult your hospital for a definition of the range of ages for pediatric deaths.

$$\frac{\text{Total number of autopsies performed on pediatric deaths for a period}}{\text{Total number of pediatric deaths for this period}} \times 100$$

Calculating Emergency Department Autopsy Rates

$$\frac{\text{Total number of autopsies performed on ED deaths for a period}}{\text{Total number of deaths occurring in the ED for this period}} \times 100$$

Calculating the Crude Birth Rate

$$\frac{\text{Number of live births in a given period}}{\text{Mid-interval population in that period}} \times 1000$$

Calculating the Fertility Rate

$$\frac{\text{Number of live births in a given period}}{\text{Population of females from ages 15 to 44}} \times 1000$$

Calculating the Out-of-Wedlock Birth Ratio

$$\frac{\text{Out-of-wedlock live births}}{\text{Mid-interval population}} \times 1000$$

Calculating the Teenage Pregnancy Rate

$$\frac{\text{Number of live births among females ages 15 to 19}}{\text{Mid-interval female population from the same ages}} \times 1000$$

Calculating Low Birth Weight (LBW) Births

Low birth weight (LBW) is considered to be less than 2500 grams (about 5 pounds 8 ounces) and is a measure of neonatal health.

$$\frac{\text{Number of low birth weight (LBW) babies}}{\text{Total live births}} \times 1000$$

Calculating the Crude Death Rate

$$\frac{\text{Total number of deaths}}{\text{Mid-interval population}} \times 1000$$

Calculating the Age-specific Death Rate

$$\frac{\text{Total deaths in a specific age group}}{\text{Mid-interval population of the same age group}} \times 1000$$

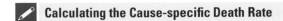

Calculating the Cause-specific Death Rate

$$\frac{\text{Deaths due to a specific cause}}{\text{Mid-interval population for a given period}} \times 100{,}000$$

Calculating Maternal Mortality Rate

$$\frac{\text{Total maternal deaths}}{\text{Total live births}} \times 100{,}000$$

Calculating the Abortion Rate: Method 1

$$\frac{\text{Legal induced abortions}}{\text{Mid-interval population of women aged 15 to 44}} \times 1000$$

Calculating the Abortion Rate: Method 2

$$\frac{\text{Legal induced abortions}}{\text{Total live births}} \times 1000$$

Calculating the Late Fetal Mortality Rate

$$\frac{\text{Number of late fetal deaths}}{\text{Live births + late fetal deaths (stillbirths)}} \times 1000$$

Calculating the Early Neonatal Mortality Rate

$$\frac{\text{Number of early neonatal (birth to less than 7 days) deaths}}{\text{Live births}} \times 1000$$

Calculating the Neonatal Mortality Rate

$$\frac{\text{Number of newborn deaths ages birth to less than 28 days}}{\text{Live births}} \times 1000$$

Calculating the Postnatal Mortality Rate

$$\frac{\text{Number of infant deaths from 28 days to 1 year}}{\text{Live births}} \times 1000$$

Calculating the Perinatal Mortality Rate

$$\frac{\text{Number of late fetal deaths } + \text{ early neonatal deaths}}{\text{Live births } + \text{ late fetal deaths}} \times 1000$$

Calculating the Infant Mortality Rate

The infant mortality rate includes deaths of infants from birth through the first year of life.

$$\frac{\text{Number of infant deaths birth to 1 year}}{\text{Live births}} \times 1000$$

Calculating Incidence

$$\frac{\text{Reported new cases of a disease for period}}{\text{Mid-interval population}} \times 1000 \text{ or more}$$

Calculating Prevalence

$$\frac{\text{Reported new and existing cases of a disease for period}}{\text{Population during that time period}} \times 1000 \text{ or more}$$

Calculating Productivity Based on Completed Work

$$\text{Productivity} = \frac{\text{Completed Work}}{\text{Time Period}}$$

Calculating Unit Cost

$$\text{Unit Cost} = \frac{\text{Annual Compensation}}{\text{Annual Productivity}}$$

Calculating Staff Levels Based on Volume

$$\text{FTEs} = \frac{\text{Volume of Dictation}}{\text{Productivity}}$$

Calculating ROI Costs

$$\text{ROI cost} = \frac{\text{Salary of ROI staff}}{\text{Number of pages or number of requests}}$$

Calculating Case Mix Index

$$\text{Case Mix Index} = \frac{\text{Total Weights for a Period of Time}}{\text{Total Patients for a Period of Time}}$$

Calculating the Payback Period

$$\text{Payback period} = \frac{\text{Cost of equipment}}{\text{Estimated cash inflow}}$$

Calculating Return on Investment

$$\text{Return on investment} = \frac{\text{Average annual savings}}{\text{Purchase price}} \times 100$$

ANSWERS TO EXERCISES, BRIEF CASES, AND REVIEW QUESTIONS

CHAPTER 1: Introduction to Statistical Terms and Concepts in Health Data Management

Exercises

Exercise 1-1. Numbers at Work

1. Health care statistics directly or indirectly facilitate patient care.
2. b

Exercise 1-2. Uses and Users of Health Care Data

1. b
2. secondary

Exercise 1-3

1. b

Exercise 1-4. Health Care Data Classifications

1. False: the hospital names/facilities are nominal data.
2. d
3. c

Exercise 1-5. Obtaining and Comparing Health Care Data

1. d
2. b

Brief Cases

Running the Numbers

1. a
2. c

Checking the Codes

Sasha recognizes that the format of these codes is incorrect. She knows the format for the ICD-10-PCS codes requires at least four characters.

Review Questions

1. The data consists largely of the administrative, financial, and clinical data collected by the facility or clinicians. Examples of data items in health care are as varied as patient age, sex, marital status, or diagnosis. Because of the complex and inclusive

nature of health care data, it would also include the salaries of nurses, the cost of medical office space, the outcome of medical procedures, and the results of diagnostic testing.

2. b

3. a

4. a

5. b

6. Data sets standardize which group of data elements are collected, which allows the comparison of two different facilities or the performance of the same facility over time.

CHAPTER 2: Basic Math Concepts, Central Tendency, and Dispersion

Exercises
Exercise 2-1. Fractions

1. a. $\dfrac{12}{8} = 1\dfrac{1}{2}$ b. $\dfrac{5}{2} = 2\dfrac{1}{2}$ c. $\dfrac{144}{12} = 12$

2. a. $3\dfrac{3}{8} = \dfrac{27}{8}$ b. $13\dfrac{1}{2} = \dfrac{27}{2}$ c. $7\dfrac{5}{16} = \dfrac{117}{16}$

3. a. $\dfrac{2}{8} = \dfrac{1}{4}$ b. $\dfrac{50}{100} = \dfrac{1}{2}$ c. $\dfrac{75}{1000} = \dfrac{3}{40}$ d. $\dfrac{12}{144} = \dfrac{1}{12}$

   e. $\dfrac{6}{36} = \dfrac{1}{6}$

4. a. $\dfrac{1}{8} + \dfrac{7}{12} = \dfrac{17}{24}$ b. $\dfrac{7}{8} - \dfrac{1}{16} = \dfrac{13}{16}$ c. $\dfrac{1}{2} - \dfrac{1}{5} = \dfrac{3}{10}$

   d. $\dfrac{2}{3} + 1\dfrac{1}{3} = 2$ e. $3\dfrac{5}{8} + 7\dfrac{3}{4} = 11\dfrac{3}{8}$

Exercise 2-2. Decimals

1. Convert the following fractions to decimals:

   a. $\dfrac{3}{8} = 0.375$ b. $13\dfrac{1}{2} = 13.5$ c. $7\dfrac{5}{16} = 7.3125$

   d. $\dfrac{1}{160} = 0.00625$ e. $\dfrac{60}{10000} = 0.006$

2. hundredths

3. millionths

4. a. 0.09513999: tenths = 0.1; hundredths = 0.10; thousandths = 0.95
   b. 0.551031: tenths = 0.6; hundredths = 0.55; thousandths = 0.551
   c. 1.342809: tenths = 1.3; hundredths = 1.34; thousandths = 1.343

Exercise 2-3. Percentages

1. a. 10/50 = 20%
   b. 49/100 = 49%
   c. 17/1000 = 1.7%
   d. 14/16 = 87.5%
   e. 1810/2000 = 90.5%

2. a. 1% = 0.01
   b. 10% = 0.10
   c. 47% = 0.47
   d. 0.5% = 0.005

3. Convert the following to the simplest fraction:

   a. $0.5 = \dfrac{1}{2}$
   b. $0.98 = \dfrac{49}{50}$
   c. $0.333333333 = \dfrac{1}{3}$

   d. $1.75 = 1\dfrac{3}{4}$
   e. $90\% = \dfrac{9}{10}$
   f. $25\% = \dfrac{1}{4}$

Exercise 2-4. Ratio, Rate, and Proportion

1. 7.5 minutes:1 chart

2. 4

3. 2:5

Exercise 2-5. Volume, Frequency, and Frequency Distribution

1. The absolute frequency is the total; 25 + 16 = 41. The relative frequency of males is 60.98%, and for females, it is 39.02%. The simplest form of the boy:girl ratio is 25:16.

2. The 11 classes would be as follows: 25,000-30,000; 30,001-35,000; 35,001-40,000; 40,001-45,000; 45,001-50,000; 50,001-55,000; 55,001-60,000; 60,001-65,000; 65,001-70,000; 70,001-75,000; and 75,001-80,000.

Exercise 2-6. Measures of Central Tendency

1. 3.25

2. a. 9.25
   b. 10
   c. 10
   d. Removing the values 3 and 15 give us an adjusted mean of 9.3.

Brief Cases
Working with Fractions

Asian-American: $\dfrac{10}{120} \div 10 = \dfrac{1}{12}$

Latino or Hispanic: $\dfrac{35}{120} \div 5 = \dfrac{7}{24}$

African-American: $\dfrac{15}{120} \div 15 = \dfrac{1}{8}$

Finding Mean, Median, and Mode

In this example, the mode (most frequently appearing observation) is 2 days AND 3 days since the most frequent number of discharges is 7—observed in both lengths of stay. Note that the mean is 2.76 (58 total days divided by 21 discharges), and the median is 3 (observation #11 is 3 days). So, our measures of central tendency are roughly in agreement. In general, newborns this week stayed, on average, about 3 days.

Review Questions

1. a. $\dfrac{18}{8} = 2\dfrac{1}{4}$ b. $\dfrac{21}{2} = 10\dfrac{1}{2}$ c. $\dfrac{14}{12} = 1\dfrac{1}{6}$

2. a. $\dfrac{33}{66} = \dfrac{1}{2}$ b. $\dfrac{5}{100} = \dfrac{1}{20}$ c. $\dfrac{750}{1000} = \dfrac{3}{4}$

3. a. $\dfrac{1}{12} + \dfrac{7}{12} = \dfrac{2}{3}$ b. $\dfrac{1}{8} - \dfrac{2}{3} = -\dfrac{13}{24}$ c. $4\dfrac{1}{2} - 3\dfrac{1}{5} = 1\dfrac{3}{10}$

4. a. $\dfrac{1}{8} = 0.125$ b. $\dfrac{1}{22} = 0.0\overline{45}$ c. $\dfrac{14}{12} = 1.1\overline{6}$

5. a. $0.09513999 = 0.1; 0.10$
   b. $0.551001 = 0.6; 0.55$
   c. $22.7399 = 22.7; 22.74$
   d. $1.1733 = 1.2$

6. a. $55\% = 0.55$
   b. $17\% = 0.17$
   c. $1156\% = 11.56$
   d. $0.034 = 3.4\%$
   e. $0.78 = 78\%$
   f. $1.11 = 111\%$

7. 107.67, or about 108 students

8. 0.025 g

9. 3657 g

10. 8

11. 15

12. The mean in the average, useful to indicate the number of times something usually occurs, or the most usual amount. Extreme values or outliers can affect the mean, making it less reliable to indicate the usual amount.

13. The absolute frequency is 136. Male RF = 36.76%; Female RF 63.24%. The simplest ratio is 25:43.

14. There would be 15 class widths of $5,000 and four of $20,000.

15. Mean: 28.52; Median: 22; Mode: 19; Range: 58; Variance: 217.9696; SD: 14.91368362

CHAPTER 3: Data Presentation

Exercises

Exercise 3-1. Tables

1. Column header

2. Frequency table

3. A pivot table works by automatically extracting the information you want to see and summarizing the information in a smaller, separate table.

Brief Cases

Checking Your Work

Let us start from the top.

1. The title is okay, but it is missing the date range. That would certainly be important!

2. Each of the box heads should be treated the same; he forgot to make the percentage of cumulative frequency bold like the others.

3. We might expect that we would not have any patients between the ages of 91 to 100 who were treated for this disorder, but Prasad should have put zeros in these cells, not left them blank.

4. According to the table, patients between the ages of 81 to 90 make up 8.0% of these cases. The relative frequency of 1/125 is 0.8%, not 8.0%!

5. While the contents of cells may be centered, right justified, or left justified, the table should be consistent. The frequencies 3 and 7 should be moved to the left.

6. This frequency distribution is not exhaustive! All the data you have should fit into all the categories you have. If you look closely, you will see that the classes skipped the age 30.

7. It is not mutually exclusive either, meaning no piece of data could fit into two separate categories. Unfortunately, 10-year-old patients could fit in one of two classes in this distribution.

8. While it might seem evident that exactly 40% of the patients in the bottom two bins comprise the total, we do not know for sure unless it is written as 40.0. This ensures all the values have the same amount of *significant figures*.

9. Last, are these class widths an effective way to understand the data? Since 80% of the treatments are for patients under the age of 20, more detail may be helpful. For example, if we broke the classes into intervals of 3 years, we might find that 78% of all treatments were for patients younger than 0 to 15 years of age, with those 16 to 18 and 19 to 21 accounting for just 3% of the total. This means physicians should not expect to treat too many patients older than 15, but that information is lost in the table as Prasad presented it.

Using Graphs

The first is a display of the comparison of the dollars owed between the different payers for each hospital, while the second shows a comparison of the percentage owed by the different payers for each hospital.

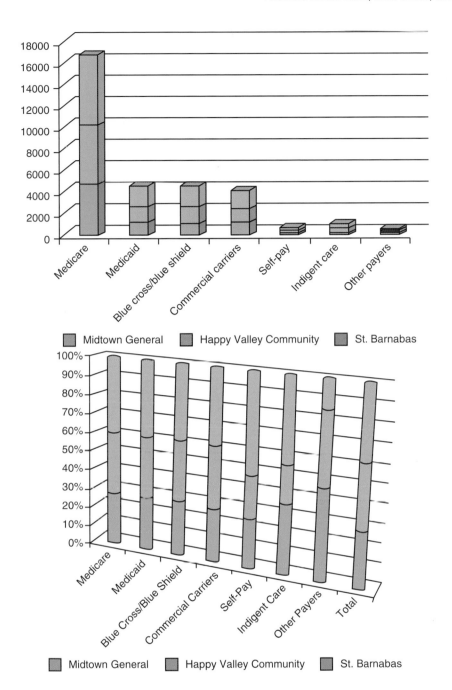

Review Questions

1. The table appearance can vary, but your layout might look like the following:

TABLE 1. Acme Home Health Nursing by Language, January–March, 20XX

	LANGUAGE SPOKEN		
Month	**Spanish**	**English**	**Total**
January	25	75	**100**
February	10	82	**92**
March	17	90	**107**
Total	**52**	**247**	**299**

2. The charts should look as follows:

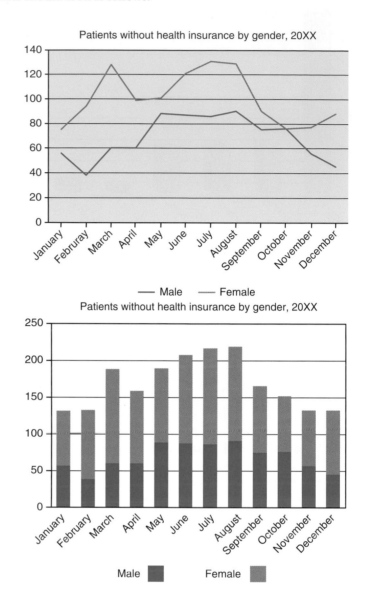

3. histogram

CHAPTER 4: Administrative Data

Exercises

Exercise 4-1. Outpatient Calculations

Physician	Visit Total Wk 1	Visit Total Wk 2	Visit Total Wk 3	Visit Total Wk 4	Physician Visit Avg	4-Week Range
Andrews	32	41	26	27	126/4 = 31.5	15
Basile	14	19	22	45	100/4 = 25	31
Chambers	31	34	32	31	128/4 = 32	3
Dahl	25	8	16	25	74/4 = 18.5	17
Edwards	27	14	16	23	80/4 = 20	13
Totals	129	116	112	151	508/4 = 127	39
Weekly average	129/5 = 25.8	116/5 = 23.2	112/5 = 22.4	151/5 = 30.2	508/20 = 25.4	30.2−22.4 = 7.8
Weekly physician range	32−14 = 18	41−8 = 33	32−16 = 16	45−23 = 22	89/4 = 22.25	33−16 = 17

1. Dr. Chambers had the highest volume of patients this month and averaged the most encounters per week.

2. Dr. Basile had the widest range of encounters this month, and Dr. Chambers had the narrowest.

3. Weekly average = 25.4. Edwards' average = 20; (25.4 – 20 = 5.4). Dr. Edwards saw 5 (rounded from 5.4) fewer patients per week on average than the physician group as a whole.

Exercise 4-2. Inpatient Census

1. a

2. It would be inappropriate to place a newborn in an adult-sized bed and impossible to put an adult in a bassinet.

3. 16

4. a. 157
   b. 12
   c. 158

Exercise 4-3. Occupancy

Use the table below to answer the following questions.

	Month	IPSDs	Bed Count	Occupancy %
1st Quarter	January	5500	200	0.887097
	February	5789	200	1.03375
	March	4700	200	0.758065
2nd Quarter	April	4920	200	0.82
	May	4000	150	0.860215
	June	3780	150	0.84
3rd Quarter	July	3991	150	0.85828
	August	3921	150	0.843226
	September	3568	150	0.792889
4th Quarter	October	3666	150	0.788387
	November	5000	200	0.833333
	December	5524	200	0.890968

1. Bed count days: 6200; Occupancy rate: 76%

2. 103%

3. 89%

4. 84%

5. 85%

Exercise 4-4. Length of Stay

Calculate the individual LOS for each of the following patients:

1. 3

2. 1

3. 1

4. 5

5. 30

6. 62

7. $102 \ (3+1+1+5+30+62)$

8. $102/6 = 17$

9. ALOS for adults and children: $700/125 = 5.6$; ALOS for newborns: $51/17 = 3$

10. a. 61.9%
    b. 2.2
    c. 2.224

Brief Cases
Counting Patients

To find the bed count days, we multiply the number of beds that are set up, staffed, and ready for patients each day (200) by the number of days in the period of time we are looking at (30). In this month, the hospital has 6000 bed count days. When we are looking for the occupancy rate, the bed count days goes in the denominator. She would set up her calculation like this:

$$\frac{4250 \text{ IPSDs}}{6000 \text{ bed count days}} = 0.708333 \times 100 = 71\%$$

The numerator is the total number of IPSDs times 100, divided by the total possible number of beds that could have been filled in that same time period. In September, the occupancy rate at Michael's hospital was a bit low, at 71%. The hospital used 71% of the resources it made available.

Comparing Utilization

Happy Valley Hospital 2015

ALOS A&C	42,555 discharge days/14,501 discharges = 2.934 rounded to 2.93 ALOS for adults and children
ALOS NB	1899 discharge days/899 discharges = 2.032 rounded to 2.03 ALOS for newborns
ADC A&C	40,866 IPSDs/365 = 111.961 rounded to 111.96 ADC A&C
ADC NB	1537 IPSDs/365 = 4.210 ADC NB
%Occupancy A&C	$40,866 \times 100/125 \times 365 = 4,086,600/45,625 = 89.569$ rounded to 89.60%
%Occupancy NB	$1537 \times 100/5 \times 365 = 153,700/1825 = 84.219$ rounded to 84.22%

St. Barnabas 2015

ALOS A&C	29,452/8960 = 3.287 rounded to 3.29
ALOS NB	1242/1002 = 1.239 rounded to 1.24
ADC A&C	24,245/365 = 66.424 rounded to 66.42
ADC NB	1234/365 = 3.380 rounded to 3.38
%Occ A&C	$24,245 \times 100/365 \times 90 = 2424500/32850 = 73.805$ rounded to 73. 81%
%Occ NB	$1234 \times 100/365 \times 5 = 123400/1825 = 67.616$ rounded to 67.62%

Midtown General 2015

ALOS A&C	35,500/9600 = 3.697 rounded to 3.70 days
ALOS NB	1501/905 = 1.658 rounded to 1.66 days
ADC A&C	36011/365 = 98.660 rounded to 98.66 patients
ADC NB	425/365 = 11.643 rounded to 11.64 newborns
%Occ A&C	$36011 \times 100/250 \times 365 = 3601100/91250 = 39.464$ rounded to 39.46%
%Occ NB	$4250 \times 100/25 \times 365 = 425000/9125 = 46.575$ rounded to 46.58%

The tables and charts should look as follows:

	% Occupancy A&C	% Occupancy NB
Happy Valley	89.6	84.22
St. Barnabas	73.81	67.62
Midtown General	39.46	46.58

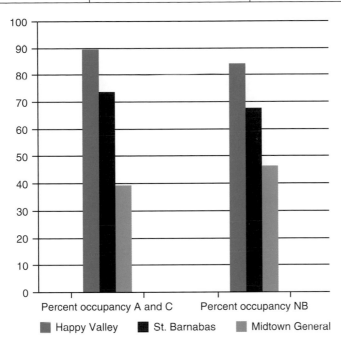

Review Questions

1. Outpatients are those who are to be treated within the same calendar day. A physician's office, the hospital emergency department, diagnostic imaging and laboratory centers, along with same-day (ambulatory) surgery centers are all examples of outpatient care. Inpatients stay overnight for at least one night in acute care hospitals, nursing homes, and other long-term care facilities.

2. A patient could be counted twice (or not at all) as they move from one unit to another.

3. Census: A&C 94, NB 4; IPSDs: A&C 95, NB 4

4. While the census shows how full the hospital is at one particular time during a day, the total IPSDs show how much work the hospital has done in that 24-hour period.

5. a. 248
   b. 5
   c. 89%

6. The occupancy % indicates how full the facility is.

7.

	Adults and Children	Newborns
Bed count days	4650	310
Occupancy	77%	40%
ALOS	7.43	3.88
Direct bed turnover rate	2.96	3.2
Indirect bed turnover rate to the thousandths place	3.213	3.196

8. LOA days are added to discharge days but not IPSDs.

CHAPTER 5: Clinical Facility Data

Exercises

Exercise 5-1. Morbidity Rates

1. patient discharges

2. 134

3. 10%

4. $97 \times 100/3017 = 3.215$ rounded to 3%

5. $513 \times 100/6824 = 7.517$ rounded to 8%

6. $97 \times 100/431 = 22.505$ rounded to 23%

Exercise 5-2. Consultation Rates

1. $815 \times 100/9743 = 8.364$ rounded to 8%

2. $2409 \times 100/9743 = 24.725$ rounded to 25%

Exercise 5-3. Obstetric Rates

1. $(7+4) \times 100/856 + (7+4) = 1.268$ rounded to 1.3%

2. $42 \times 100/167 = 25.149$ rounded to 25%

3. $3 \times 100/42 = 7.142$ rounded to 7%

4. $5 \times 100/317 = 1.577$ rounded to 1.58%

5. $3 \times 100/317 = 0.946$ rounded to 0.95%

Exercise 5-4. Mortality Rates

1. Gross: $43 \times 100/6372 = 0.674$ rounded to 0.67%; Net: $(43-17) \times 100/6372 - 27 = 0.252$ rounded to 0.25%

2. $17 \times 100/85 = 20\%$

3. $1 \times 100,000/1011 = 98.91$ rounded to 99/100,000 patients

Exercise 5-5. Autopsy Rates

1. ans: $2 \times 100/17 = 11.76$ rounded to 12%

2. $6 \times 100/13 = 46.15$ rounded to 46%

3. $11 \times 100/126 = 8.73$ rounded to 9%

Brief Cases

Finding the Complication Rate.

Gastric Bypass Surgery Complication: 14-Year Follow-Up

Complication	Cases	Result	Rate
Vitamin B_{12} deficiency	52	0.292135	29.21%
Incisional hernia	51	0.286517	28.65%
Depression	41	0.230337	23.03%
Staple line failure	39	0.219101	21.91%
Gastritis	24	0.134831	13.48%
Cholecystitis	19	0.106742	10.67%
Dehydration	12	0.067416	6.74%
Dilated pouch	4	0.022472	2.25%

If you calculated these results incorrectly, you may have had the number 312 in the denominator. While it is true that 312 is the total number of gastric bypass surgeries, 178 is the total number of times each of these complications could have occurred, because it is the number of patients we know about. That is, we do not have data about all 312 patients, only 178 of them. And what about the total number of cases? Why does it add up to 242, if there are only 178 patients under study? If you add the rates, why is the total more than 100%? The reason is because some of these patients reported more than one complication.

Michael's research into gastric bypass surgery resulted in mixed reviews by patients regarding their experiences with his facility. Although many of the patients had been successful in reducing their weight, lowering their blood pressure, and controlling their blood sugars, they had also experienced a number of complications that they were not happy with.

Comparing Mortality Rates

Postoperative Deaths by Procedure

Procedure	2011	2012	2013	2014	2015	Postop Mortality Rate
Coronary artery by-pass graft (CABG)	74	38	46	78	75	3.06%
Hip replacement	8	8	5	10	10	0.40%
Gastric bypass	4	11	5	0	0	0.20%
Sleeve gastrectomy	3	1	3	2	3	0.12%
Total surgeries performed	**1897**	**2232**	**2192**	**1898**	**1950**	

Finding the Autopsy Rate

	2011	2012	2013	2014	2015
IP deaths	143	179	223	301	316
IP autopsies	5	7	10	18	25
Autopsies on former patients	1	3	5	9	11
Bodies removed by MEs	3	1	4	9	8
Adjusted autopsy rate	**4.3%**	**5.5%**	**6.7%**	**9.0%**	**11.3%**

Diamonte acquired St. Barnabas 11/30/2013.

After collecting the needed data, he found that the autopsy rate did indeed spike after the enterprise acquired the academic medical center. He attached the necessary data and graph and sent them off to the COO along with the reports for the M&M conference. He glanced at the office clock and realized he would need to jog to catch his train. As he logged off and shut down his terminal, he reflected on a long, but satisfying day of work.

Review Questions

1. 9/8950 × 100 = 0.100 rounded to 0.10%

2. 3/2106 × 100 = 0.142 rounded to 0.14%

3. 2/9 × 100 = 22.2 rounded to 22%

4. 67/8950 × 100 = 0.748 rounded to 0.75%

5. 2/355 × 100 = 0.563 rounded to 0.56%

6. 42/356 × 100 = 11.699 rounded to 11.70%

7. $4/42 \times 100 = 9.52$ rounded to 9.5%

8. $2 + 3/365 + (2 + 3) \times 100 = 1.36$ rounded to 1.4%

9. $48/8950 \times 100 = 0.536$ rounded to 0.54%

10. $48 - 16/8950 - 16 \times 100 = 0.358$ rounded to 0.36%

11. $1/2099 \times 100 = 0.047$ rounded to 0.05%

12. $1/(2 + 3) \times 100 = 20\%$

13. $11 + 3/48 \times 100 = 29.1$ rounded to 29%

14. $(11 + 3)/48 - 5 \times 100 = 32.5$ rounded to 33%

15. $(11 + 3) + (1 + 3)/48 - 5 + 1 + 3 \times 100 = 38.2$ rounded to 38%

CHAPTER 6: Public Health Data

Exercises

Exercise 6-1. Types of Rates and Differences in Constants

1. Trends

2. Births, adoptions, marriages, deaths, divorces

3. Comparisons or benchmarks

4. The National Center for Health Statistics (NCHS)

5. Births

6. Morbidity

7. Mortality

8. Adjusted rate

Exercise 6-2. Natality Data

1. 13.33 rounded to 13.3/1000

2. 3.9 million/300 million 13/1000

3. $1,600,000/4$ million $\times 100 = 40\%$

4. 7.5% (300,000/4 million $\times 100$)

5. 31.8 rounded to 32/1000 women 15–44.

Exercise 6-3. Mortality Data

1. a. from birth up to 7 days of life
    b. from birth up to 28 days of life
    c. includes late fetal deaths plus the early neonatal deaths
    d. all deaths from birth up to 365 days from birth

2. Live births *or* the mid-interval population of women 15–44

3. Live births

4. a. 20–27 weeks
    b. >28 weeks

5. standardized and normalized

6. direct, indirect

7. indirect

8. a. $90,000/32,000,000 \times 1000 = 2.812$ rounded to 2.81 per 1000 population
    b. $10,000/1,800,000 \times 1000 = 5.555$ rounded to 5.56 per 1000 live births
    c. $(10,000 + 5000) \times 1000/1,800,000 = 8.333$ rounded to 8.33 per 1000 live births

d. There are two ways: $27{,}000/1{,}800{,}000 \times 1000 = 15$ ITOPs per 1000 live births *and* $27{,}000/15{,}000{,}000$ mid-interval population of women $15 - 44 \times 1000 = 1.8$ ITOPS per 1000 women 15–44

e. $75/2{,}000{,}000 \times 100{,}000 = 3.75$ maternal deaths per 100,000 obstetric admissions; $75/1{,}800{,}000 \times 100{,}000 = 4.166$ rounded to 4.17 maternal deaths per 100,000 women 15–44

f. $20{,}000 + 25{,}000/1{,}800{,}000 \times 1000 = 25$ infant deaths per 1000 live births

Brief Cases
Benchmarking Against National Rates

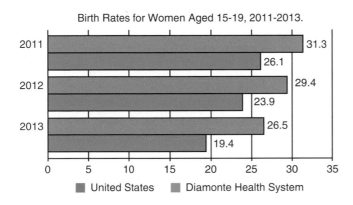

Birth Rates for Women Aged 15-19, 2011-2013.

Finding Morbidity

Cancer Site	Male	Female	Both Sexes
	AVERAGE NUMBER OF CANCERS PER YEAR IN SITES WHERE HPV IS OFTEN FOUND (HPV-ASSOCIATED CANCERS)		
Anus	106/471 = 23%	365/471 = 77%	471
Cervix	0%	100%	569
Oropharynx	277/308 = 90%	31/308 = 10%	308
Penis	100%	0%	41
Vagina	0%	100%	56
Vulva	0%	100%	452
TOTAL	424	1473	1897

Michael's hospital is seeing a lower percentage of male anal cancers (higher for female) but a higher percentage for male oropharyngeal cancers (lower for female). His analysis could be more relevant if he looked at statistics by state.

Review Questions

1. Vital statistics measure marriages, divorces, and adoptions, and births and deaths. Public health statistics do not routinely measure marriages, divorces, and adoptions.

2. True. Confounding variables are ones that may hide or change the results of a study.

3. True

4. Statistics

5. The live births to the mid-interval population

6. Adjusting rates remove the factor of differently weighted population proportions.

7. Mortality

8. Direct

9. Mortality

10. Expected

11.

Age Range	Standard Population US Pop Prop	Mortality Rate of Population of Interest (California) Crude Mortality Rate/100,000	Population of Interest Estimated Mortality Rate
0-9	0.13	62	$62 \times 0.13 = 8.06 \rightarrow 8$
10-19	0.14	27	$27 \times 0.14 = 3.78 \rightarrow 4$
20-44	0.34	95	$95 \times 0.34 = 32.3 \rightarrow 32$
45-64	0.26	503	$503 \times 0.26 = 130.78 \rightarrow 131$
65+	0.13	4007	$4007 \times 0.13 = 520.91 \rightarrow 521$

12. fertility rate and ITOP or abortion rate

13. 28

14. incidence

15. 28

16. 15

17. 28

18. perinatal

19. induced abortions

20. births

21. a. $4293/3,170,000 \times 1000 = 1.35$ rounded to 1 deaths per 1000 population
    b. $3/250,344 \times 100,000 = 1.1$ rounded to 1 per 100,000
    c. $76/4791 \times 1000 = 15.8$ rounded to 16 per 1000 live births
    d. $25 + 110/3,170,000 \times 100,000 = 4.2$ rounded to 4 per 100,000
    e. $25/3,170,000 \times 1000 = 0.7$ rounded to 1 per 100,000

CHAPTER 7: Departmental Data

Exercises

Exercise 7-1. Measure of Productivity

1. 4 FTE transcriptionists. 110 lines/hr $\times$ 8 hours a day $\times$ 20 days $= 17,600$ lines per FTE/month. $64,000/17,600 = 3.63$ rounded up to 4.

2. $3.5 \times 35 \times 50 = 6125$ charts per year. $\$17.50 \times 35$ hours a week $\times 52$ weeks $= \$31,850/$ year $\div 6125$ charts $= \$5.20$ per chart.

3. $19 \times 6 = 114/$day, $350/114 = 3.07 = 3$ FTE.

4. Coder A: 2800 ER charts coded, worked 8 hours per day, 20 days. 160 hours $= 9600$ min$/2800 = 3.43$ min/chart. Most productive.

   Coder B: 2100 ER charts coded, worked 8 hours per day, 20 days 160 hours $= 9600$ min$/2100 = 4.57$ min/chart. Least productive.

Coder C: 1100 ER charts coded, worked 4 hours per day, 20 days 80 hours = 4800 min/1100 = 4.36 min/chart.

As you can see, when the data is broken down in this manner, the HIM manager can see why the productivity standards are important!

5. $29,000/55 \times 4 \times 52 = \$29,000/11,440 = \$2.53/page$

Exercise 7-2. Reimbursement Statistics

MS-DRG	Patient Discharges	Relative Weight	Weight Total
039–Extracranial Procedures W/O CC/MCC	88	1.0452	91.9776
057–Degenerative Nervous System Disorders W/O MCC	71	0.9841	69.8711
064–Intracranial Hemorrhage or Cerebral Infarction W MCC	70	1.7417	121.9190
065–Intracranial Hemorrhage or Cerebral Infarction W CC	69	1.0776	74.3544
066–Intracranial Hemorrhage or Cerebral Infarction W/O CC/MCC	50	0.7566	37.8300
069–Transient Ischemia	50	0.6948	34.7400
074–Cranial & Peripheral Nerve Disorders W/O MCC	48	0.8786	42.1728
101–Seizures W/O MCC	46	0.7569	34.8174
149 Dysequilibrium	43	0.6184	26.5912
176–Pulmonary Embolism W/O MCC	42	0.9891	41.5422
177–Respiratory Infections & Inflammations W MCC	37	1.9934	73.7558
178–Respiratory Infections & Inflammations W CC	29	1.3955	40.4695
189–Pulmonary Edema & Respiratory Failure	18	1.2184	21.9312
	661		711.9722

1. 711.9722

2. $711.9722 \div 661 = 1.0771$

3.

Month	Discharges	Total Weight	CMI
January	2331	8355.49281	3.5845
February	2646	8819.9118	3.3333
March	2100	6757.3800	3.2178
April	2191	6483.1690	2.9590
May	2520	7270.2000	2.8850
June	1946	5424.2804	2.7874
July	1806	5618.6466	3.1111
August	2520	7572.6000	3.0050
September	2800	8396.3600	2.9987
October	2408	7192.9368	2.9871
November	2877	9104.2665	3.1645
December	2863	9417.5522	3.2894

Exercise 7-3. Accreditation Statistics

1. May, June, and July

2. 330

3. 193

4. The answer is 7 in both cases.

Brief Cases

Erasing the Backlog

Trans	Avg Lines/Day	Extra Lines for Incentive Pay	Cost/Line for Normal Time	Projected Incentive Pay/Line for Additional Work	Days to Complete Additional Lines	Cost/Transcriptionist for Extra Lines (Backlog)
Aisha	1270	4375	0.12	0.18	4375/1270 = 3.4 days	$787.50
Brianna	730	4375	0.08	0.12	4375/730 = 6.0 days	$855.00
Charles	850	4375	0.08	0.12	4375/850 = 5.1 days	$855.00
Darlene	1150	4375	0.12	0.18	4375/1150 = 3.8 days	$787.50
Total	4000	17,500	X	X	X	$3285.00

$3285.00 and 3.4–6.0 days. The entire backlog would be caught up in an additional six working days at a cost of $3285.00. A savings of $390 would be realized by using their own transcriptionists.

Identifying Revenue Sources

	Initial Relative Weight	Relative Weight Change	New Relative Weight	New Total Weight	Base Rate Example (×$1100)
A = 523 patients	2.0330	15%	2.33795	1222.7478	1222.7478 × $1100 = $1,345,022.50
B = 689 patients	0.9960	18%	1.17528	809.7679	809.7679 × $1,100 = $890,744.69
C = 602 patients	1.9460	4%	2.02384	1218.3416	1218.3416 × $1100 = $1,340,175.70
D = 586 patients	1.4530	10%	1.6016	938.5376	938.5376 × $1100 = $1,032,391.30

To clarify, DRG A = 523 × 2.0330 = 1063.2590. We then increase relative weight by 15%: 2.0330 × 1.15 = 2.33,795. The new weight and new total is 523 × 2.33,795 = 1222.7478. Note that when increasing a number by a percentage, such as 15% in this case, the most efficient calculation (which saves the step of adding the increase to the original number) is to multiply the initial number by 1.15. With these adjustments, you might notice that DRG A now generates the most revenue. If the base rate for the facility is $1,100, then total payment is $1,345,022.50, even though the fewest patients are assigned this DRG.

Case Mix Investigation

CMI Averages per Quarter for Coders: 2015–2016

	First Quarter 2015	Second Quarter 2015	Third Quarter 2015	Fourth Quarter 2015	First Quarter 2016	Second Quarter 2016	Third Quarter 2016	Fourth Quarter 2016
Mary	1.2390	1.2214	1.1376	1.1689	1.2135	1.1739	1.2108	1.2594
Andrew	1.2249	1.2003	1.2121	1.1329	1.2260	1.2157	1.2241	1.1998
Joan	1.2423	1.3151	1.2971	1.2455	1.2646	1.2439	1.2876	1.2321
Frances	X	X	X	2.1943	1.9523	1.9793	1.8999	1.9247
Facility CMI Avg.	1.2354	1.2456	1.2156	1.4354	1.4141	1.4032	1.4056	1.4040

The Facility CMI equals the sum of each coder's CMI divided by 4. For the 4th quarter of 2015, the equation would look like this:

$$1.4354 = \frac{Mary + Andrew + Joan + Frances}{4} \quad or \quad \frac{1.1689 + 1.1329 + 1.2455 + x}{4}$$

Add the CMI averages for the coders, then multiple each side of the equation by four to remove the denominator:

$$4 \times 1.4354 = 3.5473 + x$$

Subtract 3.5473 from each side to isolate the unknown, Frances' average CMI for Q4 2015:

$$5.7416 - 3.5473 = 3.5473 - 3.5473 + x$$

$$2.1943 = x$$

Upon sharing the results with the coding supervisor, she learned that while the existing hospital coders worked on a mix of charts, the new coder, Frances, coded the cardiology physician group charts that were predominantly high-weighted stent placements and CABGs along with the regular hospital charts. Ana makes a mental note to thank the coding manager for explaining what could have been a suspicious possibility of upcoding.

Review Questions

1. $2080 \times 1800 = 8{,}744{,}000$ images per year. If 3 weeks are taken for vacation and holidays, then 3 weeks = 120 hours $2080 - 120 = 1960 \times 1800 = 3{,}528{,}000$. If a push rate is given of 2000 images per hour, $1960 \times 2000 = 3{,}920{,}000$ images.

2. 16 days off $\times$ 8 hours = 128 hours $1664 - 128 = 1536$ hours $\div 8 = 192$ productive days. $222{,}000/192 = 1156.25$ lines per day.

3. 60 minutes in an hour $\div$ 15 minutes per chart = 4 charts per hour, for a total of 389.5 hours to code all the records ($1558 \div 4$). Four charts per hour $\times$ 8 hours per day = 32 charts per day $\times$ 5 days = 160 charts per week $\times$ 4 weeks = 640 charts per month. $1558 \div 640 = 2.43$ FTEs, or two full-time and one part-time coder.

4. Per day, 3 charts/hour $\times$ 8 hours = 24 charts coded per day. Per week, 24 charts $\times$ 5 days = 120 charts per week. Per month, this would be $120 \times 4 = 480$. $1802/480 = 3.75$ FTEs, which is three full-time coders and one three-quarter-time coder.

5. $12 \text{ hours} \times 60 \text{ minutes} = 720/20 = 36$ requests per day.

6. $2915.2882/1567 = 1.8604$, so this was calculated incorrectly, and the reported CMI of 2.1326 is incorrect. The Happy Valley CMI of 1.8604 is higher than that of St. Barnabus. This could be due to more intense type of services offered at our facility, or perhaps we recently instituted a clinical documentation improvement program that allowed us to capture more diagnoses for coding and higher DRG rates.

7. $1802 + 1959 + 1972 = 5733/3 = 1911$ average discharges. 1911×0.5 delinquency allowable $= 955.5 = 956$ charts allowed to be delinquent to stay in compliance. For H&Ps, Joint Commission and Medicare require 100% compliance, but facilities are given a little bit of leeway in this goal. Our facility has allowed a 2% delinquent rate, which means $1911 \times 0.02 = 38.22$ or 39 H&Ps can be delinquent, and we are still compliant.

CHAPTER 8: Financial Data

Exercises
Exercise 8-1. Capital Budget

1. $\$500 \times 12 = \$6000$. $\$6000/\$18,000 \times 100 = 33.3\%$

2. $\$6000/\$250 = 24$ months

3. $\$8800/4 = \$2200$

Exercise 8-2. Operational budget

1. fixed

2. fixed

3. $\$31,200/12 = \$2600$. $\$2600 \times 0.01 = \$26 + \$2600 = \$2626$; $\$2600 \times 0.05 = \$130 + 2600 = \$2730$. $\$2730 + \$2600 = \$5356$

Brief Case
Preparing an RFP

1. $300,000 \times 0.05 = 15,000$. A 5% return rate represents a 95% accuracy rate.

2. $300,000 \times 1.5 = 4500$; $100 - 98.5 = 1.5$. Your facility requires that 98.5% of claims are accurate the first time they are submitted; this allows for a 1.5% error (return) rate.

3. $15,000 \times 0.20 = 3000$. We are only looking at the number of returned claims, and if we reduce the number of claims by 80%, then we are still expecting that 20% of the claims will be returned.

4. $\$106,000/\$39,000 = 2.7$ years

5. $\$39,000 \times 100/\$106,000 = 36.8\%$

Review Questions

1. Operational budgets include routine expenditures, planning for payroll, office supplies, equipment leases, and maintenance contracts, and even travel, dues, and education expenses for employees. Capital budget expenditures are large purchases, such as equipment, computers and other technology, and new shelving or office furniture.

2. Proposal 1:

$$\text{Payback period} = \frac{\$3,800}{\$1,800} = 2.1111 \text{ years or 2 years and 1.3 months}$$

Proposal 2:

$$\text{Payback period} = \frac{\$4,100}{\$1,200} = 3.4167 \text{ years or 3 years and 5 months}$$

Reliable Copier Company's payback period is quicker.

3.

	ScanTron	ScanTek	Scans 'R' Us
Price	$7900	$8400	$6500
Savings per month	$225	$275	$180
ROI	$225 × 12 = $2700	$275 × 12 = $3300	$180 × 12 = $2160
	$2700/$7900 = 34%	$3300/$8400 = 39%	$2160/$6500 = 33%

4.

Item	Budget	Actual	$Var	%Var
Payroll	$1,560,000	$1,555,555	~~$4555~~ $4445	0.28%
Outsourcing	$5000	$10,750	($5750)	~~115%~~ (15%)
Supplies	$3500	$3000	$500	~~12.4%~~ 14.3%
AHIMA dues and credentials	$2220	$2405	~~($85)~~ ($185)	(8.3%)
Equipment depreciation	$3750	$3750	0	~~100%~~ 0%
Equipment lease	$7200	$6000	$1200	~~0.16%~~ 16%
Equipment rental	$700	$1400	$700	~~(100%)~~ 100%

CHAPTER 9: Scrubbing and Mapping Data

Exercises
Exercise 9-1. Data Quality

1. Data granularity
2. Data currency
3. Data comprehensiveness
4. A data dictionary is a list of details that describes each field in a database, and it contains those specific details as to how the information must be recorded. In this way, it ensures the data is consistent, comprehensive, relevant, and recorded with the proper level of granularity.

Exercise 9-2. Data Scrubbing

1. Foreign-key constraint
2. Unique constraint
3. Data-type constraint

4. Range constraint

5. Set member constraint

6. Mandatory constraint

Exercise 9-3. Data Mapping

1. Source

2. Heuristics

3. Equivalence

4. Target

Brief Cases
Using Quality Data

1. Consistency

2. Accuracy and granularity

Scrubbing Your Data

Last Name	First Name	Zip Code
Anton	Mark	**5899**
Bahar	Allen	58991
Crawford	Sarah	**58991-2344**
Darden	Tawanna	**589,999**
Endee	Robert	**5899!**
Frick	David	58,923
George	Ivory	**58,832**
Hu	Dallas	58992-33
Iwasaki	Thomas	058,999
Jurawski	Geoffrey	**58999-**

Data Dictionary
Patient Demographics

Name	Definition	Size	Type	Example
FNAME	Patient's first name	15 Characters	Alphabetic	Geoffrey
LNAME	Patient's last name	15 Characters	Alphabetic	Jurawski
ZIP	Patient's zip code	5 Characters	Numeric	58831

Mapping Data

Disease/Disorder	ICD-9-CM	ICD-10-CM
Rubella, NOS	056.9	B06.9
Rubeola, NOS	055.9	B05.9
Mumps, without complication	072.9	B26.9
Tuberculosis of lung, infiltrative, unspecified	011.00	A15.0
Syphilis, unspecified	097.9	A53.9
Rabies, unspecified	071	A82.9
Varicella, NOS	052.9	B01.9
Poliomyelitis, acute paralytic, unspecified	045.10	A80.30
Diphtheria, unspecified	032.9	A36.9
Pertussis, unspecified	033.9	A37.90
Ebola virus disease	065.8	A98.4

Review Questions

1. data currency
2. data consistency
3. data comprehensiveness
4. data harmonization
5. data accuracy
6. heuristics
7. foreign-key constraint
8. range
9. target
10. set-membership
11. data consistency

CHAPTER 10: Predicting Data

Exercises

Exercise 10-1. Samples, Populations, and Probability

1. probability
2. non-probability
3. sample
4. probability sampling
5. convenience
6. systematic random sampling
7. stratified random sample
8. 32%
9. 7/sqrt of 25 = 7/5 = 1.4

   For 2 SD 1.4*2 = + or −2.8 for SE, so confidence interval is 74.2–79.8.

Exercise 10-2. Hypothesis Testing

1. Null
2. Type I
3. Alternate
4. Type II
5. Significance

Brief Cases

Selecting a Sample

1. C
2. A
3. B
4. D

Testing a Hypothesis

Aiko should reject the null. This is a positive correlation.

Review Questions

1. descriptive

2. inferential statistics

3. probability

4. standard error

5. central limit theorem (CLT)

6. population

7. sampling bias

8. non-probability sampling

9. cluster sampling

10. simple random

11. systematic

12. stratified

13. convenience

14. judgment sampling

15. quota sampling

16. snowball

17. The confidence level is the degree to which you can be reasonably sure that another researcher would be assured of a similar study result. It is calculated as the percentage of the population that will yield an observation within a stated range. The significance level also shows how reliable (repeatable) the results are, but it is a number set ahead of time used to either accept or reject the null hypothesis.

18. SE = 0.9/sqrt of 81

    0.9/9 = 0.1

    SE = 0.1

    For 99% confidence level, (3 sd) 0.1 * 3 = + or −0.3.

    Confidence interval is 6.3 − 0.3 = 6.0 to 6.3 + 0.3 = 6.6.

    6.0 − 6.6.

19. Setting up a null and alternate hypothesis

20. Confidence interval

21. Null

22. Type I

23. Type II

24. a. inferential

    b. population

    c. probability

    d. stratified random sample

    e. null hypothesis

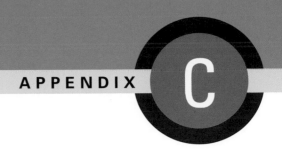

APPENDIX C

ABBREVIATION LIST

A&C	Adults and Children
A&D	Admitted and Discharged Same Day
AAP	American Academy of Pediatrics
ADC	Average Daily Census
AHIMA	American Health Information Management Association
AHRQ	Agency for Healthcare Research and Quality
ALOS	Average Length of Stay
AMA	Against Medical Advice
AP-DRG	All Patient Diagnosis-Related Groups
APR-DRG	All Patient Refined Diagnosis-Related Groups
ARRA	The American Recovery and Reinvestment Act
ASC	Ambulatory Surgery Center
CABG	Coronary Artery Bypass Graft
CARF	Commission on Accreditation of Rehabilitation Facilities
CC	Comorbidity or Complication
CDC	Centers for Disease Control and Prevention
CEO	Chief Executive Officer
CERT	Comprehensive Error Rate Testing
CFO	Chief Financial Officer
CIED	Cardiac Implantable Electronic Device
CLABSI	Central Line-Associated Bloodstream Infection
CLT	Central Limit Theorem
CMI	Case Mix Index
CMS	Centers for Medicare and Medicaid Services
COO	Chief Operating Officer
CS	Cesarean Section
CT	Computed Tomography
DEEDS	Data Elements for Emergency Department Systems
DHHS	Department of Health and Human Services
DOA	Dead on Arrival
DOB	Date of Birth
DRG	Diagnosis-Related Groups
DQM	Data Quality Model
ED	Emergency Department
EHR	Electronic Health Record
FTE	Full-Time Equivalent
FY	Fiscal Year
GAD	Generalized Anxiety Disorder
GEM	Generalized Equivalence Mapping
H&P	History and Physical
HAC	Hospital-Acquired Condition
HAI	Hospital-Acquired Infection
HEDIS	Healthcare Effectiveness Data and Information Set

HHS	Department of Health and Human Services
HIM	Health Information Management
HIMSS	Health Information Management Systems Society
HIPAA	Health Insurance Portability and Accountability Act
HIT	Health Information Technology
HITECH	Health Information Technology for Economic and Clinical Health Act
HPV	Human Papillomavirus
HR	Human Resources
ICD-10-CM	International Classification of Diseases, Tenth Revision, Clinical Modification
ICD-10	International Classification of Diseases, Tenth Revision
ICD-10-PCS	International Classification of Diseases, Tenth Revision, Procedural Coding System
ICD-9-CM	International Classification of Diseases, Ninth Revision, Clinical Modification
ICD-9	International Classification of Diseases, Ninth Revision
ICD	International Classification of Diseases
ICU	Intensive Care Unit
IPSD	Inpatient Service Day
ITOP	Induced Termination of Pregnancy
LBW	Low Birth Weight
LOA	Leave of Absence
LOS	Length of Stay
LTC	Long-Term Care
LTCH-PPS	Long-Term Care Hospital Prospective Payment System
M&M	Morbidity and Mortality
MA	Medical Assistant
MAC	Medicare Administrative Contractor
MCC	Major Comorbidity or Complication
MDS	Minimum Data Set
ME	Medical Examiner
MIC	Medicaid Integrity Contractor
MPI	Master Patient Index
MMR	Maternal Mortality Rate
MRI	Magnetic Resonance Imaging
MS	Medical Severity
NB	Newborn
NCDB	National Cancer Database
NCHS	National Center for Health Statistics
NCQA	National Committee For Quality Assurance
NIAHO	National Integrated Accreditation for Healthcare Organizations
NICU	Neonatal Intensive Care Unit
NIH	National Institutes of Health
NVSS	National Vital Statistics System
OASIS	Outcome and Assessment Information Set
POA	Present on Admission
PPM	Policy and Procedure Manual
PPO	Preferred Provider Organization
PPS	Prospective Payment System
PUB	Peptic Ulcer Bleeding
RFP	Request for Proposal

ROI	Release of Information
ROI	Return on Investment
RW	Relative Weight
SNF	Skilled Nursing Facility
SMR	Standardized Mortality Rate
TB	Tuberculosis
TJC	The Joint Commission
UACDS	Uniform Ambulatory Care Data Set
UHDDS	Uniform Hospital Discharge Data Set
WHO	World Health Organization
UTI	Urinary Tract Infection
VAP	Ventilator-Acquired Pneumonia
VBAC	Vaginal Birth After Cesarean Section
ZPIC	Zone Program Integrity Contractor

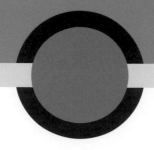

GLOSSARY

A

Abortion rate The rate of legal induced abortions within a population, also called the *induced termination of pregnancy (ITOP) rate.*

Accrual accounting An accounting method in which income and expenses are recorded when they are incurred, regardless of when the money is actually exchanged.

Adjusted rate A rate comparing the number of events (births, deaths, diseases, etc.) among populations with different demographic makeups (such as age, race, or gender) as if the two populations had the same makeup.

Alternative hypothesis The relationship between two populations expected by a data analyst.

Amortization A fixed payment schedule of principal and interest over the life of a loan.

Autopsy An examination of the body after death to either determine or confirm the cause of death.

Average daily census The total number of inpatient service days for a period divided by the days in the period.

Average Length of Stay (ALOS) The total number of discharge days for a group of patients being studied, then divided by the number of discharges in the group.

B

Bar chart A graphic display of data in which the values of variables are represented by the height or length of lines or rectangles; also called a bar graph.

Bar graph A graphic display of data in which the values of variables are represented by the height or length of lines or rectangles; also called a bar chart.

Base rate A standardized dollar amount used with an individual diagnosis-related group (DRG) to determine payment.

Bassinet count The actual number of bassinets that a hospital has staffed, equipped, and otherwise made available for occupancy by newborns for each specific operating day.

Bed count The actual number of beds that a hospital has staffed, equipped, and otherwise made available for occupancy by patients for each specific operating day.

Benchmarking The process of comparing one's results to standards or references.

Business intelligence The application of knowledge to make decisions.

C

Capital budget Money set aside for larger purchases, usually over a certain dollar amount, whose use will span multiple fiscal years.

Case mix index (CMI) The arithmetic average (mean) of the relative diagnosis-related group weights of all health care cases in a given period.

Cash flow The balance of money in and money out of the department.

Census The number of patients who occupy certain beds at a uniform time every day.

Central limit theorem (CLT) The mathematical rule stating that the observations of a sample will be distributed normally if the sample is large enough.

Class A group of values in a frequency distribution.

Complication An adverse event that happens to a patient after admission to the hospital that causes an increase in the length of stay by at least one day, in 75% of the patients.

Confidence level The percentage of the population that will yield an answer within a stated range.

Confounding variable An extra factor that masks the real relationship of occurrence or event to the population at risk for the event.

Consultation The formal request by a physician for the professional opinion or services of another health care professional, usually another physician, in caring for a patient.

Contingency table A table with two variables; also called a cross-tabulation.

Continuous data Data on a scale in which numbers have values in between the whole numbers.

Cross-tabulation A table with two variables; also called a contingency table.

Crude rate A rate comparing the number of events (births, deaths, diseases, etc.) to the entire population at risk for the event.

D

Data Items, observations, or raw facts.

Data accuracy A data quality characteristic ensuring data are correct, valid, and free from errors.

Data analytics The inspection and evaluation of groups of data using statistics to answer questions and develop conclusions.

Data comprehensiveness A data quality characteristic ensuring all required data are collected.

Data consistency A data quality characteristic ensuring data are reliable and the same.

Data constraints Rules that limit the type of data that can be entered into a field.

Data dictionary A list of details that describe each field in a database.

Data enhancement The activity of adding information by checking against a validated database.

Data harmonization The process of formatting all data items in a similar manner.

Data mapping The process of matching elements between distinct data sets.

Data scrubbing The process of making data useful for analysis. Also called *data cleansing*.

Data set A standard group of elements collected so that they can be compared with similar data.

Decimal A fraction with a denominator based on the number 10.

Delinquent record count The number of records not completed within a specific time frame, such as within 30 days of discharge.

Depreciation The loss of value over time due to wear from use and obsolescence.

Descriptive statistics The analytical activities and calculations performed to explain what *is* or what *was*.

Device days The number of patients using a device for a particular number of days.

Diagnosis-related group (DRG) A collection of health care descriptions organized into statistically similar categories.

Discharge days The number of days a patient spends in the hospital.

Dispersion The spread of the data.

E

Encounter A patient's interaction with a health care provider to receive services; a unit of measure for the volume of ambulatory care services provided.

Epidemiology The study of the occurrences, causes, and patterns of health conditions.

F

Fetal death The un-induced death of a fetus before extraction from the mother.

Fixed costs Expenses in the operational budget that do not change on a monthly basis.

Fraction A number expressed as a part of a whole.

Frequency The total number of occurrences of a value.

Frequency distribution The organization of data into tabular format using mutually exclusive classes and frequencies.

Frequency table A tabular display showing how often an observation appears in each class of a frequency distribution.

H

Health care–associated infection (HAI) An infection developed during the course of treatment.

Histograms Graphic displays of frequency distributions.

Hospital-acquired condition (HAC) Disease or disorder that occurs after a patient has been admitted to a health care facility.

I

Incidence rate The number of new cases of a disease/disorder divided by the population at risk times a constant of 100,000.

Induced termination of pregnancy (ITOP) rate The rate of legal induced abortions within a population. Also called the *abortion rate.*

Inferential statistics Statistics used to make generalizations about a population from a sample, a smaller part of the population.

Inferential statistics The study of using mathematical models to *predict* future events.

Information Data that has been organized to give it context and meaning.

Inpatient service day (IPSD) A measure of the use of hospital services representing the care provided to one inpatient during a 24-hour period.

Interval level data A type of quantitative data without a natural zero, in which the values may be added or subtracted but multiplying and dividing them has no meaning.

K

Knowledge The conclusion arrived at by using information to determine a truth.

L

Leave of Absence (LOA) days The time a patient spends outside the facility.

Length of Stay (LOS) The duration of an inpatient visit, measure in whole days; the number of whole days between the inpatient's admission and discharge.

Line graphs A graphic display of data connecting coordinates with a line, useful for showing trends over time.

M

Master patient index (MPI) A system containing a list of patients who have received care at the health care facility and their encounter information, often used to correlate the patient with the file identification.

Mean The sum of the values divided by the total number of observations.

Median The middle value of an ordered array of data.

Mid-interval population The size of the population at the midpoint of a period of time.

Miscarriage A fetal death before 20 weeks' gestation.

Mode The most frequently occurring observation in a set of data.

Morbidity A disease or illness.

Mortality Death

Mortality rate Death rate

N

Natality Birth rate

Nominal level data A type of qualitative data without a mathematical relationship or order among observations.

Non-probability sampling A sample selection method that does not seek to avoid bias and in which the selection is not done randomly.

Null hypothesis A statement that there is no relationship between the specified populations.

O

Observation bed A type of bed for a patient who may require care overnight but whose condition does not yet require an actual admission.

Occupancy It is a ratio of the number of occupied beds to the number of available beds.

Operational budget Costs related to the operation of the department, such as payroll, utilities, and supplies.

Ordinal level data A type of nominal data in which the observations have an ordered value.

Outlier An extreme value in a set of data.

P

p value The probability of mistakenly rejecting the null hypothesis when it is in fact true.

Payback period The amount of time it will take for the savings or revenues generated by a purchase to pay for the purchase.

Percentage The number of times a thing occurs out of 100.

Pictogram A graphic display using icons to represent numbers.

Pie charts A graphic presentation of data showing data categories as percentages of a whole.

Pivot table An Excel tool that extracts data from a large table into a smaller table.

Population An entire group; every actual or potential element, item, or individual under study.

Precision The significant figures, or the number of digits to the right of a decimal.

Prevalence rate The number of new and existing cases of a disease/disorder in a population divided by the population at risk times a constant of 100,000.

Primary data In health care, items that are obtained directly from the patient record and which specifically identify that patient.

Probability The likelihood that an event will happen.

Probability sampling A sample selection method that seeks to avoid bias by choosing a random selection.

Productivity standard An expectation of the amount of work performed.

Proportion The relation of four quantities in two equal ratios, where the first quantity divided by the second equals the third divided by the fourth.

Prospective payment system (PPS) A system used by payers, primarily the Centers for Medicare and Medicaid Services (CMS), for reimbursing acute care facilities on the basis of statistical analysis of health care data.

Public health statistics Statistics that describe the wellbeing of populations, such as an entire city, state, or country.

Push rate A productivity standard slightly higher than the average or usual amount of work completed.

Q

Qualitative data Observations without a numerical value that can be sorted or counted into categories.

Quantitative data Numeric data

Quotient The result of division.

R

Range The difference between the lowest and highest (or highest and lowest) observation.

Rate A value in relation to a different unit.

Ratio A comparison of two or more numbers using the same unit of measurement.

Ratio level data A type of quantitative data with a meaningful, natural zero in its order.

Relative frequency The observed frequency of a value divided by the absolute frequency (the total).

Relative weight (RW) A number assigned yearly by the Centers for Medicare and Medicaid Services (CMS) that is applied to each diagnosis-related group (DRG) and used to calculate reimbursement; this number represents the comparative difference in the use of resources by patients in each DRG.

Return on investment The percentage of the capital expenditure recovered each year.

Rolling quarterly average The average of the previous three months.

Rounding The process of reducing the number of digits in a number to make it easier to use.

S

Sample A subset of the population that has been selected using a particular sampling method.

Sampling bias A distortion of the true nature of the population, caused by non-random sampling.

Sampling error The possibility that the mean of the sample is different than the mean of the population and therefore not representative of the entire population.

Scatter diagram A type of chart that uses coordinates to help visualize suspected cause and effect relationships between independent and dependent variables.

Secondary data Summarized or abstracted items that may or may not be patient identifiable.

Significance A measure of the reliability of an observed effect.

Source In data mapping, the original data set mapped to the target.

Specific rate A rate comparing the number of events (births, deaths, diseases, etc.) within a demographic subset of a population (people of a certain age, race, sex, etc.) to the entire population at risk for the event.

Standard deviation A measure of variance showing how different the observations are from the mean.

Standard Error (SE) The difference between the means of samples of a population.

Statistics The scientific application of mathematical principles to the collection, analysis, interpretation, and presentation of numerical data.

Swing bed A type of bed that may be used for either acute or long-term care.

T

Target In data mapping, the data set to which the source is mapped.

Type I error The rejection of the null hypothesis when it is actually true.

Type II error The acceptance of the null hypothesis when it is actually false.

V

Value The count or measurement of the observation.

Variable An item or characteristic that is measured or counted.

Variable costs Expenses in the operational budget that change month-to-month based on the volume of activity.

Variance A deviation from the projected spending in the budget.

Vital statistics Public health data collected through birth certificates, death certificates, and other data-gathering tools.

Volume The count of an activity or value.

X

X-axis The horizontal (left-to-right) axis.

Y

Y-axis The vertical axis, showing the frequency of the dependent variable.

INDEX

Page numbers followed by "*b*", "*t*", and "*f*" refer to boxes, tables, and figures respectively.

CONVERTING UNITS

METRIC AND STANDARD UNIT CONVERSIONS

Moving among units within the metric system works the same whether you are measuring length in meters, weight in grams, or volume in liters. The prefix *kilo* always means 1000 of the basic unit, and the prefix *milli* always means one-thousandth (1/1000) of the basic unit. There are 1000 grams (g) in one kilogram (kg). A milliliter (mL) is 1/1000 of a liter. *Centi* means 100, so there are 100 centimeters in a meter, or 1 centimeter is 1/100 of a meter.

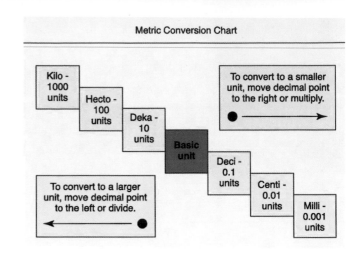

Metric Conversion Chart

Kilo - 1000 units
Hecto - 100 units
Deka - 10 units
Basic unit
Deci - 0.1 units
Centi - 0.01 units
Milli - 0.001 units

To convert to a smaller unit, move decimal point to the right or multiply.

To convert to a larger unit, move decimal point to the left or divide.

Units of Mass

10 milligrams (mg) = 1 centigram (cg)
10 centigrams = 1 decigram (dg) = 100 milligrams
10 decigrams = 1 gram (g) = 1000 milligrams
10 grams = 1 dekagram (dag)
10 dekagrams = 1 hectogram (hg) = 100 grams
10 hectograms = 1 kilogram (kg) = 1000 grams
1000 kilograms = 1 megagram (Mg) or 1 metric ton (t)

Units of Length

10 millimeters (mm) = 1 centimeter (cm)
10 centimeters = 1 decimeter (dm) = 100 millimeters
10 decimeters = 1 meter (m) = 1000 millimeters
10 meters = 1 dekameter (dam)
10 dekameters = 1 hectometer (hm) = 100 meters
10 hectometers = 1 kilometer (km) = 1000 meters

Units of Liquid Volume

10 milliliters (mL) = 1 centiliter (cL)
10 centiliters = 1 deciliter (dL) = 100 milliliters
10 deciliters = 1 liter (L) = 1000 milliliters
10 liters = 1 dekaliter (daL)
10 dekaliters = 1 hectoliter (hL) = 100 liters
10 hectoliters = 1 kiloliter (kL) = 1000 liters

Units of Volume

1000 cubic millimeters (mm^3) = 1 cubic centimeter (cm^3)
1000 cubic centimeters = 1 cubic decimeter (dm^3)
             = 1,000,000 cubic millimeters
1000 cubic decimeters = 1 cubic meter (m^3)
             = 1,000,000 cubic centimeters
             = 1,000,000,000 cubic millimeters